Information Management for Health Professions

The Health Information Management Series

Merida L. Johns

Shirley Anderson
Series Editor

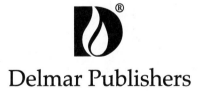

Delmar Publishers

an International Thomson Publishing company **I(T)P**®

Albany • Bonn • Boston • Cincinnati • Detroit • London • Madrid
Melbourne • Mexico City • New York • Pacific Grove • Paris • San Francisco
Singapore • Tokyo • Toronto • Washington

NOTICE TO THE READER

Cover Design: Brucie Rosch

Publishing Team:
Publisher: Susan Simpfenderfer
Acquisitions Editor: Marlene Pratt
Developmental Editor: Jill Rembetski
Project Editor: William Trudell

Art and Design Coordinator: Rich Killar
Production Coordinator: Cathleen Berry
Editorial Assistant: Sarah Holle
Marketing Manager: Darryl L. Caron

COPYRIGHT © 1997
By Delmar Publishers
a division of International Thomson Publishing Inc.

The ITP logo is a trademark under license

Printed in the United States of America

For more information, contact:

Delmar Publishers
3 Columbia Circle, Box 15015
Albany, New York 12212-5015

International Thomson Publishing Europe
Berkshire House 168-173
High Holborn
London, WC1V7AA
England

Thomas Nelson Australia
102 Dodds Street
South Melbourne, 3205
Victoria, Australia

Nelson Canada
1120 Birchmount Road
Scarborough, Ontario
Canada M1K 5G4

International Thomson Editores
Campos Eliseos 385, Piso 7
Col Polanco
11560 Mexico D F Mexico

International Thomson Publishing Gmbh
Königswinterer Strasse 418
53227 Bonn
Germany

International Thomson Publishing Asia
221 Henderson Road #05-10
Henderson Building
Singapore 0315

International Thomson Publishing - Japan
Hirakawacho Kyowa Building, 3F
2-2-1 Hirakawacho
Chiyoda-ku, 102 Tokyo
Japan

2 3 4 5 6 7 8 9 10 XXX 02 01 00 99 98 97

Library of Congress Cataloging-in-Publication Data

Johns, Merida L.
 Information management for health professions / Merida L. Johns.
  p. cm. — (The Health information management series)
 Includes bibliographical references and index.
  ISBN 0-8273-5949-7 (alk. paper)
  1. Medical informatics. 2. Information resources management.
 I. Title. II. Series.
 R858.J66 1996
 610'.285—dc20   96-18463
                               CIP

Delmar Publishers' Online Services

To access Delmar on the World Wide Web, point your browser to:
http://www.delmar.com/delmar.html
To access through Gopher: gopher://gopher.delmar.com
(Delmar Online is part of "thomson.com", an internet site with information on more than 30 publishers of the International Thomson Publishing organization.)
For information on our products and services:
email: info@delmar.com
or call 800-347-7707

Dedicated to my father, Edgar C. Boetani
1904–1996

Contents

Preface   xi

Introduction   xvii

Chapter 1: **A Model of Practice for Health Information Management**   1

Definitions of Health Information Management   3
  Traditional Definitions of Information Management   3
  Traditional Roles of Medical Record Professionals   5
  Requirements for Role Change   6
  The Health Information Manager as an Information Broker   7

Model of Practice   9
  Information Engineering Domain   10
  Information Retrieval Domain   12

Information Analysis   13
  Policy Development   14

The Successful Health Information Manager   14

Chapter 2: **Concepts of Health Information Management**   18

Defining an Information System   20
  Information System Concepts   21
  Information System Components   26
  Information System Processes   27
  Categories of Information Systems   29

Information Systems and the Organization   31
  Strategic Nature of Information Systems   31
  Levels of Organizational Decision Making   32
  The Life Cycle of Information Systems in the Organization   34
  Managing the Information Resource   38

Impact of Information Systems Technology on the
Organization   42

The Importance of Systems Thinking   46

Chapter 3:   Information Systems in Health Care   50

History of Information Systems in Health Care   51
Distinctions between Data, Information, and Knowledge   52
Evolution of Information Systems in Health Care   54

Current Applications and Trends in Health-Care Information
Systems   59
Clinical Applications and Systems   59
Administrative and Management Applications   65

Current Trends in Health Information Systems   68
Clinical Information Systems   69
Administrative Information Systems   70
Management of the Information Resource and Standards
Development   70
The Virtual Health-Care Information System   71

Chapter 4:   Strategic Planning for Information Systems   75

Health-Care Organizational Strategic Planning Process   78
Organizing Resources   78
Environmental and Internal Analyses   80
Generating Options and Developing and Enterprise Strategy   87

Information System Strategic Planning   88
Information System Strategic Planning Methods   88
Developing a Customized Information Systems Planning
Methodology   91

The Health Information Manager's Role in
Strategic IS Planning   96

Chapter 5:   Design and Development of Information Systems   100

Traditional Systems Development Life Cycle   101
New Approaches and New Tools   104
Development of the Enterprise Information Model   104

Computer-Aided Software Engineering Tools   *105*

Rapid Application Development Tools   *107*

Joint Application Design   *108*

Use of New Approaches for Analysis and Design   **108**

Data Modeling   *108*

A Definition of Data Modeling   *111*

Categories of Data Models   *113*

Content of a Conceptual or Business Data Model   *114*

Data Modeling Methods and Styles   *116*

Steps in the Data Modeling Process   *119*

Developing Data Model Diagrams   **128**

Martin Information Engineering Style   *129*

A Sample Data Modeling Diagram Project   *137*

Translation of the Conceptual Data Model to a Physical Data Model   *144*

Chapter 6:   **Database Management Concepts**   **148**

Database Management Concepts   **152**

Files, Records, and Fields   *152*

File versus Database Processing   *154*

Database Structure Models   *159*

Database Management System Functions   **168**

Storing, Retrieving, and Updating Functions   *169*

Data Dictionary   *170*

User Interface   *171*

Transaction Support   *171*

Data Integrity Services   *172*

Concurrent Processing Controls   *173*

Recovery Services   *174*

Authorization Controls   *175*

Functions of Data and Database Administrators   **176**

Data Administrator Roles   *177*

Database Administrator Functions   *188*

Chapter 7:   Managing Data Quality   192

The Origins of Data Quality   195

Characteristics of Data Quality   196

Determining the Quality of Data   200

Determining Data Quality Requirements   201

Measuring and Tracking Data Quality   204

Analyzing Results of Monitoring and Tracking   206

Improving Processes That Use and Create Data   206

Implementing Information Systems Data Control Features   207

Chapter 8:   Data Retrieval and Analysis   211

Retrieval and Manipulation of Data   213

Structured Query Language   213

Query by Example   225

Analyzing Data   228

Analysis Design   228

Sample Case Data   230

Fundamental Concepts   230

Descriptive Measures   232

Determining Significance and Group Differences   242

Data Presentation Techniques   244

Graphing Data   244

Use of Computer Statistical Packages   253

Chapter 9   Security, Audit, and Control of Health Data   256

Privacy and Confidentiality of Health Data   258

Legislative Protection of Privacy   260

Security Fundamentals   262

Protecting Informational Privacy   263

Protecting Data Integrity   266

Ensuring Data Availability   267

Conclusion   267

Establishing a Security Program   268

Components of a Security Program   *270*
Conclusion   *274*

Risk Analysis and Management   **274**
Risk Analysis   *275*
Sample Risk Assessment   *280*
Development of Countermeasures   *282*

Prevention and Control Countermeasures   **283**
Personnel Security   *284*
Physical Security   *286*
Hardware Security   *288*
Software Security   *289*
Communications Security   *293*
Conclusion   *294*

Business Continuity Planning   **294**
Goals of the Business Continuity Plan   *295*
Development and Content of the Business Continuity Plan   *295*

In Conclusion   **303**

Glossary   **305**

Index   **311**

Preface

Health information management can be defined as "the effective collection, analysis, and dissemination of quality data to support individual, organizational, and social decisions related to disease prevention and patient care, effectiveness of care, reimbursement and payment, planning, research and policy analysis, regulation and accreditation" (Cassidy and Brodnick, 1991). This definition has been applied by the American Health Information Management Association (formerly the American Medical Record Association) to describe the functional shift in paradigm from that of archivist to that of information manager and broker. While the definition provides a global perspective of tasks, there are still questions that arise regarding the roles within this new paradigm of practice.

The purpose of this text is to provide a schema for role definition by illustrating the constructs proposed in the information management model of practice that was developed by Johns (1991). These constructs relate to data capture, data analysis, data retrieval, and information dissemination. The book expands each of these constructs by adopting the perspective that information must be managed as a resource with emphasis on concepts of information ownership, structure, content, and appropriateness. A professional model of practice characterizing the health information manager as a broker of information services is developed and explored throughout the text.

In Chapter 1, a model of health information management practice is presented. This model develops the theme of managing information as a resource and deals with practical and theoretical constructs related to the health information manager as a broker of information services. These services consist of four domains of practice: information engineering, information retrieval, information analysis, and policy development. This theme continues throughout the text as a basis for comparison and development of skills in managing information as a resource.

Chapter 2 orients the student to the importance of information in health-care delivery. The chapter presents basic concepts of information systems and information management.

Chapter 3 builds on the concepts in Chapter 2 and presents a history of information systems in health care. The chapter culminates with a discussion of current trends and the need for a view of a virtual health information system.

Chapter 4 launches the detailed exploration of the four domains of health information practice. This chapter begins with the first function of information engineering—that of strategic planning for information systems. The full potential of information systems cannot be recognized unless they support the strategic goals of the organization. Thus, the foundations for successful development and deployment of information systems is grounded in the integration of business and information systems strategic planning. Principles and concepts underlying business strategic planning are presented along with elements critical to the information systems planning process.

Chapter 5 continues with the study of the information engineering domain. This chapter focuses on the elements and methodologies of conceptual data modeling on an enterprise-wide basis. This function, along with data administration responsibilities, is one of the most important information engineering functions performed by the health information manager.

Chapter 6 continues with the examination of information engineering activities. This chapter focuses on the concepts associated with a database environment and contrasts these to the traditional file processing environment. The importance of a database approach to data storage and retrieval for today's health-care enterprise is discussed. The functions associated with systems to manage databases are explored along with managerial tasks of a data administrator. The position of data administrator is an emerging job opportunity and one in which health information managers should take a proactive role.

Chapter 7 introduces the importance of data quality management. With a tradition of maintaining separate business unit systems and files, transforming to database systems has uncovered many quality problems in today's health-care enterprise data. This chapter focuses on the concepts associated with data quality and provides an overview of strategy for managing the data quality in a health-care organization.

Chapter 8 introduces the domains of information retrieval and analysis. An overview of two data manipulation languages is presented for data extraction from a database environment. Retrieval of appropriate data is the first step in any data analysis project and is often one that presents significant barriers. Data analysis is presented from the perspective of a three-step process: identification of the questions for study, identification of the variables necessary to study the questions, and selection of appropriate statistical methods and techniques to support robust analyses. The chapter concludes with a review of data presentation techniques.

Chapter 9 provides an overview of data security, audit, and control from policy and procedural perspectives. Emphasis is placed on introducing the learner to a basic knowledge and skill set that would form the foundation for a role as chief security officer in a health-care facility.

Use of This Book in the Academic Curriculum

This textbook can be successfully used in associate, baccalaureate, and master-degree programs in health information management. At the associate level, the text can function as the primary source for introducing learners to the emerging roles in health information management. At this level, the text provides sufficient breadth and depth necessary for a global understanding of the new milieu of health information management practice and concepts associated with database approaches to health data storage, retrieval, and management of data quality.

For the baccalaureate and master's level, this text provides an excellent medium for introducing the fundamentals of health information management practice in the age of the computer-based patient record. It presents in simple terms the concepts associated with emerging new health information management practice areas. It is ideal for providing foundational knowledge in key health-care information systems and management concepts and practices that can be augmented later in the curriculum through other coursework in these domains.

The text can also be used successfully as an adjunct to courses in other health-care-related fields to prepare health professionals in the functions of health information management. Among these are curricula in allied health professions, public health, nursing informatics, and health services administration.

Features

The book provides the following features to assist the learner in developing knowledge and skills:

- Learning Objectives placed at the front of each chapter. The objectives serve as a guide to the learner in identifying the key concepts of the chapter.
- Key Terms placed at the front of each chapter. These terms are defined at the end of the text in the Glossary.
- Review Questions at the end of each chapter aimed at higher levels of cognitive reasoning and analysis.
- Suggested Enrichment Activities at the end of each chapter. These activities are designed to allow the student an opportunity to investigate how theory and concepts are being applied in the real-world work setting.

Acknowledgments

I wish to extend my appreciation to a number of individuals without whose help this text would not have been possible. First, to Russell Johns for his support, counsel, and advice. His input contributed clarity in development of several passages of the manuscript and his continued encouragement provided me with the motivation to see the work through to the end. Second, to the reviewers of this text who provided thoughtful guidance and confirmation that I was on the right track.

Shirley Anderson, PhD, RRA
Professor
Department of Health Information Management
St. Louis University
St. Louis, MO

Melanie Brodnik, PhD, RRA
Director and Assistant Professor
Health Information Management and Systems Division
The Ohio State University
Columbus, OH

Nancy Coffman, MS, RRA
Allied Health
Indiana University Northwest
Gary, IN

Shirley Higgin, MEd, RRA
Program Director and Instructor
Health Information Technology
Spokane Community College
Spokane, WA

John Lynch, PhD
Director and Associate Professor
Health Information Administration Program
University of Wisconsin, Milwaukee
Milwaukee, WI

Jody Smith, MSM, RRA
Chair
Department of Health Information Management
St. Louis University
St. Louis, MO

Karen Youmans, MPA, RRA, CCS
Health Services Administration/Health Information Management
University of Central Florida
Orlando, FL

Special thanks to: Gary Davis, Captain, U.S. Air Force Medical Service Corp and graduate student in the Master of Science in Health Informatics Program at the University of Alabama at Birmingham, who assisted with the development of the data modeling diagrams; and to Terrell Herzig, also a graduate student in the Master of Science in Health Informatics Program, who assisted with the development of the QBE screens. Most sincere appreciation to series editor Shirley Anderson, whose continued confidence and support helped me to the finish line.

References

Cassidy, B., and Brodnick, M. (1991). The American Medical Record Association health information management initiative. Presentation at the Annual Meeting of the Ohio Medical Record Association, April 8, Columbus, OH.

Johns, M. L. (1991). Information management: A shifting paradigm for medical record professionals? *Journal of the American Medical Record Association, 62* (8), 55–63.

Introduction

What are the typical images that come to mind when you think about the health-care delivery process in a hospital, a clinic, an extended-care facility, or a physician's office? Probably you are thinking of health-care professionals such as physicians, nurses, therapists, and technicians assisting each other in caring for patients. Your view may also include clusters of support personnel such as receptionists, secretaries, unit clerks, housekeepers, maintenance personnel, and volunteers performing tasks that help to maintain efficient operations of the enterprise.

In addition to personnel, you might think of a variety of buildings that provide the physical room for delivery of patient care. You might be more specific in your view of physical space and conjure up images of surgical suites, delivery rooms, examination rooms, and intensive-care units. To complete your picture, you might also be thinking of the eclectic collection of equipment and supplies necessary to support the health-care delivery process; laboratory machines, respirators, radiographic equipment, monitors, and medication carts.

All of these components—personnel, facilities, and equipment—paint the picture of what is essential in the health-care delivery process. Certainly there are other aspects. There is a need for organization, capital, quality control, standardization, and cooperation. Beyond these obvious images and requirements, the basic question is, What is the glue that holds it all together? Beyond a doubt, a critical element that makes it all work is exchange of *information*. Like a spider's web, information and associated information technologies provide the essential links in supporting the function of organization, the coordination of activities, the transfer of knowledge, and the provision of care. Just as financial institutions, airlines, and government institutions cannot operate without sophisticated and coordinated information interchange, health-care delivery cannot function with-

out technologies that support information management. But like the fila-
ments in the spider's web, information infrastructures must be appropriately designed and managed in order to support health-care delivery.

Health Information Management

What is health information management? Before answering this question,
it is important to recognize that health-related information and its management can be viewed from various perspectives. The following diagram
presents several of these views.

Data Categories

- Clinical Data
- Demographic
  Data
- Financial Data
- Published
  Literature
- Research Data
- Epidemiological
  Data

Control and Managemet
of Information Resources

- Strategic Planning
- Systems Planning
- Integration of
  Information System
  Resources
- Maintenance of
  Information System
  Resources
- Policies/Procedures
  Acquisition
  Implementation
  Operation

Information Worker

- Use Information
  Resources
  Retrieve data
  Store data
  Manipulate data
  Analyze data

Information as a
Resource

- Information
  Ownership
- Information
  Structure
- Information
  Content
- Information
  Appropriateness

Perspectives of Health Information Management

One way of looking at health information management is by categories of data. Clinical information includes data that relate to direct patient care, for example, data relating to diagnostic test results, procedures, and care and treatment of the patient. Another category of health-related information is demographic data, including vital statistics about patients, health providers, and health institutions. Examples of these data are patient age, sex, and address or size, location, and average length of patient stay for a specific hospital. Financial information as it applies to various aspects of health-care delivery and cost can also be considered a component of health-related information. This information may include data relating to diagnosis-related groups (DRGs), third-party billing, and budgeting and control. Among the many categories of health-related information are published literature, and health research and epidemiological data.

Another way to view health information management is from the perspective of control and management of information resources. This functional view is often referred to as information resources management, or IRM. This perspective of health information management includes a broad range of responsibilities including strategic information systems planning, integration and maintenance of all organizational information technologies, and coordination of policies and procedures for technology acquisition, implementation, and operation.

A different view of information management is the concept of the information worker. This broad view suggests that anyone whose primary work is handling information can be viewed as an information manager. A closely related concept is that information management includes the personal management of information. Certainly in health care we can identify numerous individuals who would qualify as information workers or managers. Among these are health-care practitioners such as physicians, nurses, and therapists, and others such as medical records/health information professionals, information system specialists, medical librarians, epidemiologists, researchers, and medical communication professionals.

Besides viewing information management from the vantage of data categories, information resources management, or personal information management, another viewpoint considers managing information as a resource. The primary functions related to information management in this context deal with issues associated with information ownership, structure, content, quality, and appropriateness. This viewpoint is a critical contribution to the field for a number of reasons. First, this perspective consists of elements that are vital to the success of the other information management functions previously discussed. For instance, in order for the information worker to use and manipulate information, data must be arranged in appropriate structures that facilitate storage and retrieval. In order to promote information worker efficiency, data must be of high quality and must be supplied to the right individual at the right time. The elements of ownership, quality, content, structure, and appropriateness also support the desired outcomes of IRM. Acquisition of sophisticated computer systems and management and coordination of policies and procedures relating to information technologies cannot sufficiently compensate for poorly organized, unreliable, and inappropriate data.

Thus, the foundation for a successful information system fundamentally rests on the content, organization, reliability, and appropriateness of its data. This critical view of information management as it applies to patient-related data is examined in this text.

Chapter 1

A Model of Practice for Health Information Management

Learning Objectives

After completing this chapter, the learner should be able to:

1. Discuss the various definitions of information management and identify critical differences among them.
2. Discuss traditional roles of health information management and why these roles must change to meet today's information needs.
3. Discuss reasons for changing roles in health information management.
4. Define health information broker.
5. Identify the kinds of roles assumed by health information managers in relation to health broker tasks/activities.
6. Discuss the types of activities that might be included in various health information brokerage tasks.
7. Discuss the professional model of practice of a health information manager.

Key Terms

Data administration

Data modeling

Information broker

Information engineering

Process modeling

Strategic planning

Introduction

As discussed in the Preface, the definition of health information management has been somewhat hazy. Specifically, what tasks or functions are included under the umbrella of health information management? The answer to this question in the past has depended to a large degree on the perspective of the individual professional. However, as the pressures of health-care reform intensify the need for more and better information, there has emerged a set of functions that are crucial for ensuring the availability of quality information to health-care practitioners, administrators, researchers, and policymakers. These functions can be aligned into four domains to develop a general model of professional practice for health information management. Such a model helps to clarify the essential tasks associated with health information management in an automated environment.

Before studying the specific functions of health information management, it is important to understand the model of professional practice. To be a successful health information management professional requires not only knowing how to perform specific information management tasks but knowing how these tasks are related to each other in a systems perspective. In other words, to be successful you must know where it is that you want to go before you can actually reach your destination. Therefore, the purpose of this chapter is to help you understand your destination point— to help you understand the professional model of practice that is the underpinning of the functions of health information management.

To introduce the professional model of practice, three themes compose the first part of this chapter: (1) definitions of information management; (2) the traditional role of health information managers (i.e., medical record professionals); and (3) the requirements for changing from an archivist role to a proactive role as a broker of information services. The chapter's final section provides a new model of responsibilities for the health information manager. These responsibilities are categorized as information brokerage activities. An overview of each of these activities is presented as an introduction to more in-depth exploration in subsequent chapters.

Definitions of Health Information Management

The term *health information management* covers a broad range of skills, knowledge, and tasks. For example, health information may refer to patient educational materials, public health literature, health knowledge in published format, or data in a clinical record. Management is often associated with planning, control, and implementation.

It is important to recognize that information management means different things to different people. With such definition variety, the vision of a profession may become obscure to external stakeholders, and even to professionals themselves. Thus, the need for specificity in defining boundaries of practice becomes critical.

Traditional Definitions of Information Management

There are several different perspectives of what makes up information management. The literature provides several definitions that differ substantially depending on the perspective of the authors. For example, Synnott and Gruber (1981) identify the information management function with control and management over information resources. From their perspective, the integration of diverse disciplines, technologies, and databases is included. Achieving integration involves planning for information systems and management of both people and technology. Frequently this broad scope of information management is referred to as information resources management or IRM.

The IRM function is usually performed at an executive level within the organization. The position is commonly referred to as the chief information officer, or CIO. The CIO usually assumes a broad range of duties including organizational information systems strategic planning; integration of all organizational information technology such as data processing, office systems, and telecommunications; provision and maintenance of all information technologies; and development and coordination of policies and procedures for technology acquisition, implementation, and operation.

Information management, however, can be viewed from the perspective of information attributes rather than management functions such as planning, integration, and coordination of policies. Schneyman (1985) suggests that information management, or IM, refers to information characteristics such as information ownership, content, quality, and appropriateness. This definition suggests that IM is primarily concerned with information as an asset and therefore its intrinsic attributes must be managed effectively.

Strassman (1985) and Shortliffe and colleagues (1990) have taken the view that information management involves the personal management of information. This perspective suggests that anyone who handles information rather than physical goods is an information worker and thus an information manager. Shortliffe and colleagues, for example, state that "the practice of medicine is inextricably entwined with the management of information." That medical providers are information managers is apparent as they continually handle medical information through resources such as the hospital, medical library, patient medical records, consultation with colleagues, and memorization.

Given the variety of definitions of information management, it is no surprise that the role of the health information manager is somewhat ambiguous. To add to the confusion, many health-care professionals view their primary role as health information managers. As Johns (1991) has noted, professionals such as medical communication specialists, medical librarians, and biostatisticians all perceive that their primary tasks involve the management of health information. Thus, it is evident that the term *health information management* is not exclusive to a single profession.

Given the disparity among definitions and the differences among professional groups calling themselves health information managers, how does this text define the roles and tasks associated with health information management? An analysis must be performed that includes three critical components: (1) looking at the traditional roles assumed by medical record practitioners; (2) examining the external forces requiring changes in traditional tasks and roles; and (3) developing a model of new roles and tasks that will accommodate the information management needs of the health-care enterprise.

Traditional Roles of Medical Record Professionals

The types of tasks traditionally assumed by medical record professionals are highly quantitative and departmentally focused. A good source for identification of these tasks is the *Professional Practice Standards* (1984, 1990) published by the American Health Information Management Association (AHIMA) formerly the American Medical Record Association. A review of these standards and their accompanying evaluation mechanisms reveals that tasks of medical record practitioners involve planning, developing, and implementing systems designed to control, monitor, or track the quantity of record content, flow, storage, and retrieval or quantitative data collection on departmental personnel productivity (Johns, 1991). These traditional activities principally center around the paper medical record or clinical reports as opposed to ensuring the appropriateness, quality, timeliness, or completeness of the information itself. For example, such tasks include forms control, record tracking, incomplete record control, quantitative analysis of record content, control over release of information, and monitoring utilization of resources. As Johns point out, few tasks "specifically address issues relating to determination of the completion, significance, organization, timeliness, or accuracy of information contained in the medical record or its usefulness in decision support." In addition, traditional tasks have usually been confined to a single department (i.e., medical records department). In very few instances have tasks crossed departmental lines. Figure 1-1 provides a view of the traditional roles of health information managers.

In today's environment a new set of tasks and supporting skills is required. Because of the increasing information complexity in health-care enterprises, managers must view the world from a systems perspective, which entails a new type of problem solving. It means looking for patterns of behavior to explain situations, looking for long-term implications of trends, and trying to determine the causes of these patterns. A systems perspective views the whole enterprise *and* beyond rather than focusing primarily on a department. Thus, the health information manager must look globally for answers to problems. The focus must be interdepartmental as well as interenterprising. The types of information management tasks that will be explained later in this text are based on a foundation of systems thinking.

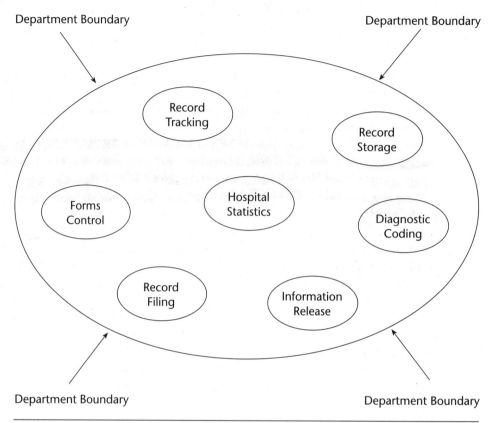

Department Boundary

Department Boundary

Department Boundary

Department Boundary

Figure 1-1. Traditional Model of Practice

Requirements for Role Change

It is a well-accepted fact that the complexity of enterprises of every type is steadily growing (Martin, 1984). Associated with this complexity is the growing intricacy of information processing. The complexity of information systems and their associated tasks has become overpowering and is frequently associated with cost. Statistics to support this opinion are abundant in the health-care industry. For example, an estimated 25 to 40 percent of a hospital's operating costs is related to information handling (Blum, 1986; Protti, 1984). The classic study by Jydstrup and Gross (1966) found that information-handling activities on a medical-surgical unit consumed 58 percent of the available time of the head nurse. Similarly, registered nurses on the same unit spent 36 percent of their time on information-handling activities. These researchers also found that, on average, 26 percent of all employee activity in a hospital is related to information handling.

The information intensiveness of health care is not only attributable to internal processes. External forces, such as accreditation requirements and federal legislation, have affected the information resources of the health-care industry. Implementation of peer review organizations and prospective payment has been labeled the most far-reaching health-care legislation since the passage of Medicare. This type of legislation demands that hospital management use analyses that previously were nonexistent or were of minor importance (Bassett, 1984). Similarly the expansion of managed care is demanding new types of information and new methods of analysis.

Technology advances have also played a role in the increase of information complexity. The 1980s and 1990s have witnessed technological advances in computer technology. With the advances, the prices of processors and storage and peripheral devices have decreased while hardware performance characteristics have increased dramatically. During the entire year of 1965, the chemistry department at Mount Sinai Hospital in New York performed 260,000 tests. After installation of the SMAC, 8,000–10,000 tests per day were being performed (Blum, 1986).

Both external and internal forces have increased health-care enterprise dependence on information to operate and manage their organizations, justify costs, prove quality, and remain competitive. These forces are depicted in Figure 1-2. The increasing information dependence has heightened the role and status of information technology and the management of information. It has also emphasized the need for transformation in information-handling roles. Thus, the traditional tasks performed by health information managers, which were primarily event driven and departmentally focused, do not work any longer in the current complex and competitive environment. An entirely new bundle of information services, called health information brokerage services, is essential to meet today's needs.

The Health Information Manager as an Information Broker

A broker acts as an agent in making contracts or sales. The broker acts as an intermediary between a client or customer and a product or service that

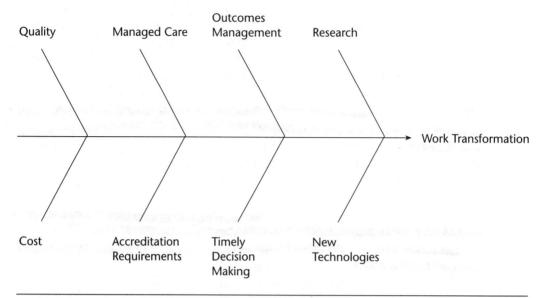

Figure 1-2. Forces Demanding Work Transformation

the customer desires. In the case of an information broker, the broker acts as an intermediary between a client and an information product or group of services. The client may desire a specific product such as the development of a decision support system, or the client may desire a certain service, such as locating a certain type of information.

In the health-care environment, the client or customer can be any number of professionals, departments, or groups. For example, the client may be a top executive who needs information about case mix within the enterprise. The client may be a physician who needs to collect research data for a clinical trial. The client may be the medicine department that needs specific display screens developed as a front end to a hospital information system or the marketing department that needs to collect and analyze data on patient satisfaction. Clients may be external to the organization, such as accrediting bodies, licensing agencies, or government organizations. In some instances, the client may be the patient who the health-care enterprise serves. It becomes evident that the client list is not exhaustive. What is apparent, however, from the list presented above is that the focus of clients' needs cross a variety of domains.

Model of Practice

Health information services can comprise a broad range of activities. For instance, information services might include operation and maintenance of physical components of an information system such as computers, wiring, printers, modems, disk drives, or tape drives. Information services may include functions associated with the design and development of software, such as systems analysis activities, programming, and software installation. Therefore, it is important that a clear definition be delineated of health information services vis-à-vis the health information manager.

Johns has noted that the tasks of a health information manager should be information based and should transcend departmental and organizational boundaries. A collection of information service tasks within the domains of data capture, data retrieval, data analysis, and information dissemination has been suggested. These functions, however, can be enhanced as shown in Figure 1-3. This professional model of practice characterizes the health information manager as a broker of information services to a multitude of clients. The information services consist of four domains of practice: (1) information engineering, (2) information retrieval, (3) information analysis, and (4) policy development. As displayed in Figure 1-3, various functions are included within each domain of practice. For example, the information engineering domain includes the functional areas of strategic planning, data administration, data modeling, and interface design. The information analysis domain includes the functional areas of decision support system (DSS) development, statistical analysis, and data presentation.

Earlier in this chapter, it was noted that the term *health information* can have a variety of meanings. Therefore, in addition to defining the type of information services provided by a health information manager, it is necessary to specify what constitutes health information. Although the health information manager will interface with many different types of information sources, most functions will focus primarily on operational and clinical data relating to episodes of patient care and to other patient or clinically related data. In this context, operational and clinical data may include data related to episodes of patient care such as results of tests and procedures, continuous quality improvement data and models (e.g., critical pathways), utilization management data, case mix data, or risk management data. Other patient and clinically related data may include patient demographics, community demographics, and epidemiological databases.

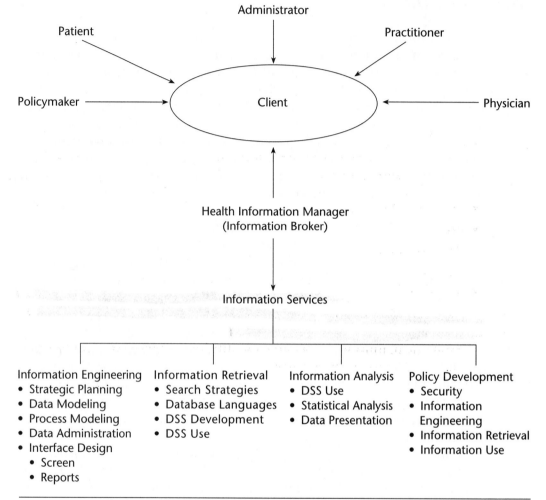

Figure 1-3. Professional Model of Practice

Information Engineering Domain

Information engineering is a collection of processes used for the planning, analysis, design, and development of information systems on an enterprisewide basis. An important concept associated with information engineering is its enterprisewide focus. In today's complex and information intensive-environment, structured and automated techniques and tools are necessary to handle the complexity of identifying information needs and designing systems to meet these needs. Formalized techniques considered in the information engineering domain include those associated with strategic planning, data modeling, process modeling, screen and report design, and development of program and data structures. Many of these techniques and tasks are very technical whereas others focus more broadly on user information needs. It is this last category of functions and techniques that will likely fall within the purview of responsibilities of the health information manager. As depicted in Figure 1-3, the normal tasks that might be assumed by the health information manager in the information engineering domain include:

- Strategic planning
- Data modeling
- Process modeling
- Data administration
- Screen design
- Report design

Strategic planning involves the identification of the goals and the critical success factors of the enterprise. These goals and critical success factors must be achieved to maintain a competitive advantage. Strategic planning from an information systems perspective is the identification of how information technology can support the critical success factors and achievement of enterprisewide goals. The result of information systems strategic planning is a high-level view of the enterprise, its functions, data, and information needs. While the techniques associated with strategic planning are usually applied to develop an enterprisewide view, the techniques can also be used to define strategic areas of opportunity for specific business areas, functions, or departments within the enterprise. Thus, the health information manager may be asked to provide strategic planning services on either an enterprisewide or business area focus. The health information manager, functioning as an information services broker, should be prepared to either participate in or facilitate the strategic planning process, particularly on a functional level. The strategic planning services offered can include techniques for identifying critical success factors and goals, determining hierarchy of goals and critical success factors, developing functional dependency diagrams, and developing entity relationship diagrams.

Data modeling is the development of a detailed logical database design. Frequently this is called the information model of the enterprise. The data model is built on information and data gathered during strategic planning. Data models provide an overview of data required for the enterprise and structures in a logical database design. It is likely that the health information manager may be asked to provide information services for the development of enterprisewide data models.

Certain techniques, such as normalization, are employed to ensure that the logical database design is stable. Because of the complexity involved in developing data models, computer-aided software engineering (CASE) tools are used in the data modeling activity. These tools assist in the development of diagrams such as data models, data flows, and program structures.

Process modeling consists of analyzing the processes of an organization, usually on a department by department basis. The functions of the department are represented in a variety of diagrams. These include decomposition diagrams, dependency diagrams, and data flow diagrams. Frequently, process modeling is performed in parallel with data modeling. As with data modeling, CASE tools are used to support the process modeling activity.

Data administration in this model of practice consists of administrative rather than technical functions associated with data and database management. Tasks are associated with planning, policy formulation, database evaluation, data dictionary management, and user education. These data administration functions are crucial steps for ensuring quality of data.

The health information manager may be called on to provide screen design and report design services. The health information manager may participate as a consultant in determining the content or the layout of screens or reports. On a more technical level, the health information manager may use CASE tools such as screen painters, report generators, or prototyping software such as VisualBasic to develop screens or report designs.

Information Retrieval Domain

Usually information retrieval is associated with providing the appropriate information to the appropriate person at the appropriate time. However, information retrieval can have a variety of meanings depending on the context or purpose for which retrieval is done. The context may be information retrieval for control or operational systems. For example, in a patient scheduling system, retrieval of information would be for operational purposes, that is, to determine the next available appointment for a clinic visit. In contrast, the context may be for use in clinical, managerial, or strategic decision making. An example of information retrieval for clinical purposes would be a listing of all clinical laboratory results for a patient for a defined period of time during an acute-care episode. Producing a tabular listing of the number of patients seen in a specific clinic over a certain period of time to determine clinic volume is an illustration of information retrieval for management decision-making purposes. The need for data on regional competitors to determine their volume of the market would be an example of information retrieval for strategic planning purposes.

Control and operational systems usually involve structured problems(clinical) requiring the same type of data over and over again. Usually information retrieval in this context is a preprogrammed, automatic process for control and operational systems. Managerial and strategic decisions, on the other hand, usually involve semistructured or ill-structured problems. The information needed to solve these problems is usually ad hoc and one of a kind and cannot be preprogrammed or automatic. Activities associated with information retrieval for managerial and strategic decision making focus on searching various information sources, development and use of decision support systems, and use of various data extraction tools. These areas will require the skills and knowledge of the information manager.

Information Analysis

The health information manager's role includes the presentation and analysis of information. Determining the type of data presentation is an important aspect of this activity. For example, in certain problem-solving situations it may be best to present data in a tabular form; in other situations it may be best to present data in a graphical form. If a manager needs to know the number of patients seen in the organization's clinic for a 1-month period, a tabular listing is appropriate. If a manager wants to know the trend of patient volume over a period of time, a graphical representation is a better choice. The way in which data are presented and represented can impact the way data are interpreted. Knowledge of the differences in presentation formats is necessary, particularly in report design. Therefore, it is important that the health information manager has a good understanding of the appropriateness of various presentation techniques.

In addition to determining presentation formats, the health information manager may be asked to provide other analytical services. These may include the statistical analysis of data or subjecting data to various decision models. To perform these services, the health information manager must be able to apply appropriate statistical techniques and use decision models. Activities within this domain may go beyond the use of statistical and decision models. Services that may also be required could include the development of decision support systems for the manager or executive. Therefore, it is important that the health information manager have a grounding in decision support system design and development.

Policy Development

The health information manager's activities include functions relating to the development of information policy. Depending on the focus of the individual job, these policies may relate specifically to information engineering, information retrieval, or information analysis activities. For example, as a data administrator, the health information manager may develop policy in regard to development of data models or the use of CASE tools. In this same capacity, the health information manager may develop policy in regard to access to sensitive data. The health information manager can also be called on to develop enterprisewide information-related policies, for example, development of release of information, password use, and other policies that would affect all employees of the enterprise.

The Successful Health Information Manager

The theoretical model of practice depicted in Figure 1-3 presents the health information manager as a broker of a variety of information services. As the figure displays, the health information manager functions as an intermediary between clients and information engineering, retrieval, analysis, and policy development services. To be successful in providing these services, the broker must have the knowledge and skills to carry out the activities associated with each of these domains of practice. However, skills and knowledge are not enough to be successful. The broker must also have clients who want the health information manager's services. Thus, the existence of these services must be known to prospective clients and the clients must recognize the value of these services. Frequently this is not the case. The health information manager must understand the need for marketing information brokerage activities.

How can marketing of services be accomplished? First, the health information manager must understand the strategic goals of the enterprise and identify ways in which information brokerage services can support these goals. For example, if the organization has a strategic goal to become a major player in the managed-care environment, the health information manager may ask to facilitate a team that identifies the information requirements needed to support this strategic goal. Second, the health information manager must know who the potential clients are in the enterprise who could benefit from brokerage services. This involves knowing what the information engineering, analysis, and retrieval needs are of departments, clinicians, managers, and executives. For example, the health information manager may know that the quality resources department has a need to collect data from a variety of enterprise databases. However, these databases are intertwined with legacy computer systems and are not integrated. The health information manager would see this situation as an information retrieval opportunity and may assist the quality resources department in the implementation of a front-end data extraction software tool. These situations exist throughout the enterprise. To turn them into opportunities entails the ability to market information services. In order for information services to add value to the organization, health information managers must view their role not only as service providers but also as marketers of these services.

Summary

- There are many different interpretations of information management. Some interpret information management with control and management over information resources. Others view it as the planning, integration, and coordination of policies associated with information itself. Still others view it as personal management of information to perform individual job tasks.

- The traditional tasks of a health information manager involved planning, development, and implementation of systems designed to control, monitor, or track paper-based medical records.
- In today's increasingly automated environment, the roles and functions of the health information manager are changing. The health information manager is a broker of information services including those services associated with information engineering, information retrieval and analysis, and information policy formulation.

Review Questions

1. Describe the changes in the role of the health information manager during the 1990s. Why have these changes occurred? What impact will these changes have on the health information profession?

2. What makes the health information management profession unique from other information-based professions? Is there a convergence between the health information management profession and other information-based professions?

Enrichment Activities

1. Review the job position advertisements in health information management journals for the 1990s. Do you see differences in the types of job positions that are advertised? What are these differences? If changes exist, do you believe that they are significant enough to indicate that the profession is undergoing change?

2. Interview a director of health information or medical record services. Through the interview determine whether or not job functions for the director have constricted or expanded during the past 3 to 5 years. Are the job functions significantly different today than 5 years ago? Why or why not is this the case?

References

American Medical Record Association (1984, 1990). *Professional practice standards.* Chicago: American Medical Record Association.

Bassett, J. G. (1984, March). Cost-per-case reimbursement: A challenge to hospital management. *Topics in Health Record Management, 4*, 1–9.

Blum, B. I. (1986). *Clinical information systems.* New York: Springer-Verlag.

Johns, M. L. (1991, August). Information management: A shifting paradigm for medical record professionals? *Journal of the American Medical Record Association, 62* (8), 53–63.

Jydstrup. R. A. & Gross, M. J. (1966, Winter). Cost of information handling hospitals. *Health Services Research*, 235–271. Cited in Blum, B. I. (1986). *Clinical information systems.* New York: Springer-Verlag.

Martin, J. (1989). *Information engineering: Book 1: Introduction.* Englewood Cliffs, NJ: Prentice-Hall.

Protti, D. J. (1984). Knowledge and skills expected of health information scientists: A sample survey of prospective employers. *Methods of Information in Medicine, 23*, 204–208.

Schneyman, A. H. (1985, Summer). Organizing information resources. *Information Management Review, 1*, 35–45.

Shortliffe, E. H., Perreault, L., Wiederhold, G., & Fagan, L. M. (eds.) (1990). *Medical informatics computer applications in health care.* Reading, MA: Addison-Wesley.

Strassman, P. A. (1985). *Information payoff: The transformation of work in the electronic age.* New York: The Free Press.

Synnott, W. R. & Gruber, W. H. (1981). *Information resource management.* New York: Wiley.

Chapter *2*

Concepts of Health Information Management

Learning Objectives

After completing this chapter, the learner should be able to:

1. Define the concept of a system.
2. Describe the characteristics of a system and relate these to an information systems example.
3. Distinguish between system elements of input, processing, and output and give health-care examples of each.
4. Describe the contribution of and interrelationships between information system components of people, work processes, data, and information technologies.
5. Differentiate between the three levels of organizational decision making and give examples of the types of decisions that might be made at each level.
6. Describe the six types of information systems and give examples of how these support administrative, financial, clinical, and research needs of a health-care enterprise.
7. Discuss the four stages of information system life cycle and how the capabilities and needs at each stage impact the organization.

8. Identify Nolan's organization life cycle stages and discuss how the management of information technologies varies in each stage.

9. Describe the concept of information resources management (IRM) and its impact on health information systems.

10. Discuss how information systems function as change agents within an organization.

Key Terms

Chief Information Officer

Decision Support Systems

Executive Information Systems

Expert Systems

Feedback

Information Resources Management

Information System

Information Systems Life Cycle

Inputs

Management Information Systems

Office Automation Systems

Organization-wide Information Systems Life Cycle

Outputs

Processing Mechanisms

System

Transaction Processing Systems

Introduction

The health information manager must have a fundamental background in systems theory and information system concepts to be effective in carrying out job roles. This entails incorporating systems thinking in solving problems related to the introduction of information systems technology into the organization. It also includes knowledge about informations system concepts, components, and processes; how information systems may impact the culture and structure of an organization; and strategies for management of the information resource. The intent of this chapter is to present the fundamentals of this essential knowledge base for the health information manager.

Defining an Information System

Before the concepts, principles, and elements relating to the content, organization, reliability, and appropriateness of data can be studied, it is important to know the components of an **information system** and how they fit in the context of the organization. The delivery of health care is built on the use of information systems. For example, when a laboratory test, such as a complete blood count (CBC), is ordered for a patient, the physician relies on an information system to communicate the request and document test results. Specifically, the physician relies on the information system to notify nursing or laboratory personnel that a specimen needs to be collected, to notify the laboratory that a CBC needs to be performed, and to document the results of the CBC in a permanent record.

The creation of a patient bill is another good example of the important role information systems play in health care. The billing department relies on several information system databases to produce a patient bill. Before a bill can be produced, the billing clerk must have information about the patient's insurance carrier; the type of insurance coverage provided to the patient; the length of stay of the patient; the type of services provided by the health-care facility; patient demographics such as name, sex, and address; the final diagnoses and procedures performed; and diagnostic and procedural codes such as ICD-9 and CPT.

In addition to patient-care providers and operational support personnel, administrators also rely on information systems. For example, the decision to add a new service by a health-care facility is dependent on the collection and analysis of information. A health-care facility may be considering adding a new type of radiology modality. However, the purchase of equipment and renovation of facilities may be extremely costly. Before making such a large investment, the administrator will rely on several types of information systems to collect and analyze data. Some of these information systems may be external to the organization such as those that provide data on community demographics or competitors. Other information systems may be internal to the organization such as those that provide information on the demographics of past patients, referrals to other institutions, treatment profiles of facility providers, and cost data. In addition to these information sources, the administrator may use a decision support system or modeling system to help make projections about the cost/benefit of such a purchase.

The above examples provide a snapshot of the types of information systems that help support the health-care delivery process. It is important to keep in mind that information systems are present in many varieties, all of which support the clinical, operational, and managerial facets of health-care delivery.

Information System Concepts

Health information managers must understand the components of information systems and how information systems affect the organization, individuals within the organization, and interested publics outside the organization. Information systems provide opportunities to improve internal operations, create competitive advantage in the marketplace, improve patient-care delivery, enhance research, and provide better service. Information system risk occurs when the systems are not well integrated, are poorly managed, or do not support the goals of the organization. In order to exploit information system opportunities and minimize threats and risks, a thorough understanding of information system components and how these relate to the organization is necessary.

System Characteristics

A **system** is a group of components that interact to accomplish a goal or an objective. A central principle of a system is that its components interact with each other through defined relationships. Through this interaction, the components are able to create something greater than the sum of their parts. In addition to defined relationships with component parts, systems must be able to function in a dynamic environment. They must be able to self-adapt or have controls that respond to a changing climate. If a system fails to accommodate the environment or if the interactions among its component parts fail, the system becomes nonfunctional and disintegrates. Thus, a system must be composed of a group of components that:

- Interact through defined relationships
- Work toward accomplishing a goal
- Self-adapt and respond to environmental changes

Figure 2-1 provides an example of the relationship of these characteristics.

An information system is composed of a group of components (people, work processes, data, and information technologies) that interact through defined relationships to accomplish a goal. Information systems must be able to adapt to environmental change. A good example of a health-related information system is an order entry system. The goal of the system is to process physician orders. The system is composed of a group of components including people (nurses, physicians, unit secretaries, laboratory personnel), data, work processes, and information technologies. Each of these components interacts through defined relationships. The people

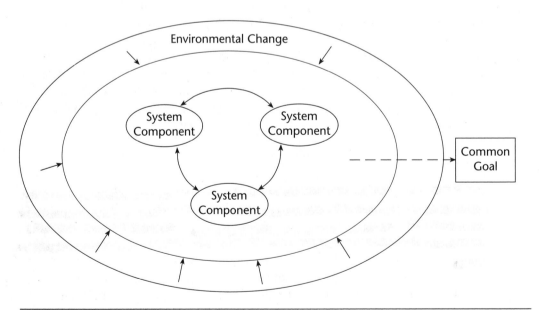

Figure 2-1. Relationship Among System Characteristics

enter orders in a predefined way through a data entry terminal (hardware) and through interaction with software. Through the predefined interactions between the hardware and software, the order is processed. The order entry system is self-adapting and able to accommodate environmental changes such as order volume. The example depicted in Figure 2-2 demonstrates the characteristics of a system as applied to an information system: component parts working in predefined relationships that can self-adapt to environmental changes to accomplish a common goal.

As the bidirectional arrows depict in Figure 2-2, at any given time there is a potential three-way interaction between all system components. People interact or are affected by work practices, data, and information technologies. Work practices affect people and may be impacted by data availability and information technologies. Information technologies may affect work practices, people, and the input, processing, or dissemination of data. Thus, we see that information components are highly interrelated. Recognizing these interrelationships is very important, since a problem with one component will likely adversely impact all other components within an information system. When information system problems arise, it is crucial that all information system components and their relationships be examined.

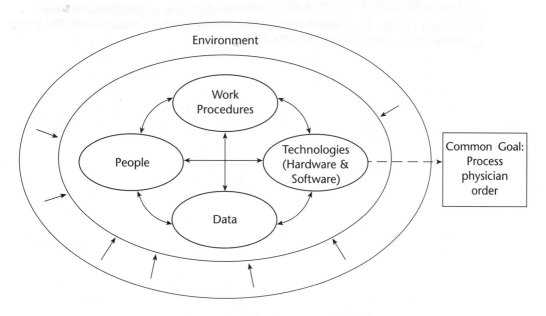

Figure 2-2. Example of an Order Entry Information System

System Elements

Systems have three principal elements: **inputs, processing mechanisms, and outputs.** Figure 2-3 depicts their simple relationship. In the order entry example given previously, inputs include physician orders such as laboratory, radiology, or pharmacy orders that are entered in a computer terminal on the patient-care unit. The orders are subjected to several processing mechanisms that check their consistency and completeness before they are routed to the appropriate department. The output of the system is a requisition for a specific type of test, procedure, or pharmaceutical. In addition to inputs, processes, and outputs, most systems also have a feedback loop. **Feedback** provided by the system influences future inputs. In the order entry example, feedback regarding nonavailability of an ordered drug in the pharmacy department inventory might be provided to the physician. In this case, the system might suggest what alternatives or substitutes are available.

Classification of Systems

Typically systems can be classified in several ways. A system may be simple or complex. It may be an open or a closed system. Systems can also be categorized as stable or dynamic and as permanent or temporary. A simple system contains few components and the relationships that exist among the components are not complex. An example of a simple information system would be an automated physician referral system. In this type of system a prospective patient may call an information number and request the names of physicians in a certain geographical area that are specialists in a specific field of practice—for instance internists or obstetricians. The system would then provide the caller with a list of physicians

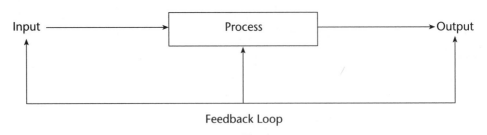

Figure 2-3. Relationship of System Elements

that meets the caller's requested parameter. The input for the system would be the caller's request. The system would process the request by searching its database for a match with the request. The output would be the list of candidate physicians.

A complex system, in contrast, has many components whose relationships are highly complicated. An example of a complex information system is an order entry system in an acute-care facility. This type of system has many (hundreds) possible inputs. These may include orders for laboratory tests, radiology exams or procedures, drug orders, physical therapy orders, dietitian orders, and so on. Relationships among the inputs and processes are likely to be complex. For example, when a drug is ordered, the system must check its patient database to determine if the patient has any noted sensitivities to the requested drug. The system would also check the current drug protocol of the patient to determine whether or not there are any potential interactions between the newly requested drug and any other drugs the patient is currently taking. The system would also check the completeness of the order, which may include checking for correct dosage, route of administration, and frequency of administration. The output of the system would be a complete drug requisition to the pharmacy.

Systems can also be categorized as open or closed. In a closed system there is no interaction with the environment. Typically, there are few closed systems. An open system interacts with its environment—that is, inputs and outputs flow beyond the boundary of the system. All living organisms are open systems because they have a high degree of interaction with their environment. Businesses, including health-care facilities, are open systems. Inputs are received from the environment (e.g., patients, raw materials) and outputs (services, products) flow back into the environment. Typically most health-care information systems can be classified as open systems. Except when information systems are totally automated, closed systems, *people* must be a contributing component. The people component of an information system will usually be involved with the three processes of input, manipulation, and output of data or information. The work practices of an organization are an important information system component. As discussed previously, work practices or procedures can affect the people component of the system and dictate data requirements or type of information technology. Work practices must be efficient and effective if an information system is to function optimally. The data component is the foundation of any information system. Data can come in a variety of types including formatted data, unformatted data (text), images, or sound. Information technologies include the hardware and software that perform the basic functions of input, process, and output.

Environmental interaction in an open system is an important concept. Such interaction between the system and the environment makes it essential that the system be self-adapting and able to respond quickly to the needs of the environment. If the system cannot perform these functions, it will become obsolete or cease to exist. A good example in the health-care arena would be the environmental factors influencing quick adaptation to the managed-care environment of the mid-1990s. Health-care systems that cannot accommodate the environmental forces will become obsolete and in many instances cease to exist.

Systems can be classified as stable or dynamic. A stable system does not accommodate or is not affected by changes in the environment. A dynamic system undergoes rapid and constant change due to changes in the environment. Since the mid-1980s, the health-care system in general has been categorized as a dynamic system. Information systems needed to support health care must be dynamic and adaptive as well.

Systems are also categorized as permanent or temporary. A permanent system will exist over a long period of time—for example, 10 years or longer. An example of an information system that could be classified as permanent is an employee payroll system. A temporary system will not be in existence for a long period of time. A temporary system may only be in existence for a few months or even less. An example of a temporary information system may be one that collects data and provides analysis for a specific research project or protocol. After the protocol is completed, the data may be maintained, but the information system itself will likely be dismantled.

Information System Components

All definitions of an information system must embody the essence of the four system characteristics that were previously presented. Thus, an information system is a group of interrelated and self-adapting components working through defined relationships to collect, process, and disseminate data and information for accomplishment of specific organizational goals. The components of an information system should be broadly interpreted. For example, information system components should be viewed to include people, work procedures, data, and information technologies (Alter, 1992).

Although organizational goals may not be specifically included in the components of an information system, they must be viewed as the driving force for the development, design, implementation, and evaluation of information systems. Each information system must be evaluated in terms of its contribution to meeting the goals of the organization.

Information System Processes

As displayed in Figure 2-3, information system processes are typically identified as input, process, and output with a feedback relationship between each element. For our purposes, we will elaborate on the processes that an information system is expected to perform.

Regarding input, we would expect that a health information system would have the capability of gathering, capturing, or collecting raw data. In a pharmacy system, for example, a physician prescription would be one input for the delivery of medication. In an operating scheduling system, a reservation request by a surgeon would be one input for assigning an operating room suite on a specific time and date. Input can take many forms. In a hospital inventory control system, the input may be the completion and submission of an requisition slip to central supply when instruments are used for an operation. Input to an automated order-entry system may be accomplished by completing designated display screens on a computer terminal, which would, in real time, input the data into the information system. Input can also include direct communication from one system to another. For example, the input to an order entry system may also feed or provide direct input into an inventory control system.

Regarding processing data, we would expect that the information system would be able to convert or manipulate raw data into some useful type of output and either store or transmit data or output. Processing or manipulation can include performing calculations, making comparisons, selecting alternative actions, or merely storing data for future use. In an inventory control system, processing may involve identifying the item that has been expended and subtracting the number of expended units from the amount currently in inventory. The output of the calculation would be stored in the inventory database. In a pharmacy order-entry system, processing may involve several calculations or comparisons. It may include a comparison of the ordered drug with the hospital formulary, comparison of the ordered drug with the patient's current drug profile, or comparison of the ordered drug with patient drug allergies. The results of any one of these comparisons may prompt the system to perform alternative actions. For example, if the ordered drug is not in the hospital formulary, the alternative action may be to determine what drug in the hospital formulary would be compatible with the ordered drug and subsequently to make a recommendation for its substitution.

Output is defined as the product produced from information system processes. The output may be the production of useful information from raw data or it may be the production of new data (transformed data) used as input into another system. Reports, documents, summaries, alerts, and decision actions are all examples of information output. Information output can be in the form of various type of media. For example, information output may be in the form of a printed paper report, or it can be an organized display of facts on a computer display screen, or an image such as a computerized axial tomography (CAT) scan.

It is important that every information system have a feedback process. Feedback can take the form of assessing outputs of system processes and determining whether or not adjustments or changes to input or processing activities are required (error or logical checks), or it can influence future inputs. In the first example of feedback, error checks based on outputs may be built into the system. For example, an output of a patient temperature of 140°F would be flagged as an error because it would not fall into the predetermined range of usual body temperature. In this case, the information system would determine that 140°F is out of range and provide feedback such as an alert or error report. The feedback would then be used by the caregiver to correct the input of the temperature to 104°F. In clinical information systems, this type of feedback is usually produced in real time so that error corrections can be made immediately.

Feedback is used to influence future inputs to the system. For example, with an outpatient scheduling system, patient appointments are scheduled on a specific date, at a specific time, and with a specific provider. When an appointment is made, the output is in the form of an appointment date and time with a provider and the appointment schedule database is adjusted to indicate that this specific time, date, and provider are not available to any other patient. This output would serve to influence any future inputs—that is, no other patient could be scheduled to make an appointment at that date and time with that provider. No information system can properly function without appropriate feedback mechanisms.

Categories of Information Systems

Information systems can be categorized by (1) the functional areas they serve, (2) the extent of structure they impose on work tasks, (3) the span across the enterprise, and (4) their purpose. Table 2-1 depicts these classifications.

A functional classification in health care may include categories of administrative, financial, clinical, and research information systems. Information systems can also be categorized by the extent of structure that they impose on work practices. In this instance, information systems can be classified as providing access to information or information tools such as in a results reporting system, or enforcement of rules or procedures such as in an automated system for application of practice guidelines and critical paths, or automation of most or all of the work such as a computerized hospital information kiosk.

Another way of classifying information systems is to view them from the perspective of their span across the enterprise. This categorization would include those systems that are used individually (word-processing package), those used across a work group (e-mail), and those used inter-organizationally (Internet). Another method for classifying information systems is by their purpose. For example, information systems can be clas-

Table 2-1.   Classifications of Information Systems

Functional Areas	Structure on Work Processes	Span Across the Enterprise	Purpose
Administrative	Access to	Individual	Transaction
Financial	information	Work group	processing
Clinical	Access to	Organization	Management
Research	information tools	Outside the	information
	Enforcement	organization	Decision
	of rules		support
			Executive
			information
			system
			Expert system
			Office automation

sified as **transaction processing systems (TPS)**, **management information systems** (MIS), **decision support systems (DSS)**, **executive information systems** (EIS), **expert systems** (ES), and **office automation systems (OAS)**.

Transaction processing systems typically collect and store data about transactions. A transaction can be defined as any business-related activity that would generate or modify data in an information system. Examples of transaction systems include admission/discharge systems, inventory control, accounts receivable, and order entry. In contrast, the focus of a management information system is to provide routine information to managers for decision making and managing the organization. Preplanned reports and documents generated by an MIS usually include summarized data from TPS. Typically these reports are used to monitor organization performance, maintain coordination of activities, or provide background information.

A decision support system is an interactive system that helps managers make decisions for semistructured or unstructured problems. Not only does a DSS provide information to the decision maker from a database, it also provides models and tools for the manipulation of data. A principal difference between an MIS and a DSS is that an MIS focuses on control and operational effectiveness (doing things right) whereas a DSS focuses on supporting the manager in making the right decision.

An executive information system is also an interactive system that helps managers access information. However, unlike a DSS, the EIS may not have the modeling capabilities to answer "what-if" queries. The EIS, however, usually has a more user-friendly interface than a DSS and allows the manager the ability to directly access databases and choose the format in which data are displayed. EIS usually provide functions for choosing between tabular or graphical data displays, provide triggers to highlight exceptional conditions or conditions out of expected range, and have the ability to control the level of detail (i.e., summary versus nonaggregated data) of information provided.

An expert system is a system that generates advice or suggests a decision in a well-defined and usually narrow area. ES consist of a knowledge base, a rule base, and an inference engine. Expert systems have been used in health care to support clinical decision making (i.e., suggest patient diagnoses), and in other fields to configure computers and interpret geological data. Office automation systems facilitate day-to-day processing and communication tasks. These systems include a broad range of tools such as word processors, spreadsheets, personal database systems, and electronic mail systems.

Information Systems and the Organization

It is well accepted that the introduction of information technology produces change and stress within an organization. The impact of information technology on the organization has been studied from various perspectives. The following sections provide insight into some of these theories.

Strategic Nature of Information Systems

The importance of organizational goals as a driving force for the design, development, implementation, and evaluation of information systems cannot be overemphasized. Too frequently, information systems are deployed that do not adequately support the work practices of the organization or organizational goals. An example of how organizational goals should guide the development of an information system is provided in the following scenario.

*I*n 1993, Community Medical Center developed a strategic plan for the enterprise that focused on developing strategies to become a viable player in a capitation environment. Community Medical Center recognized that because of several external forces, it had to change its organizational structure and work practices away from a fee-for-service environment. Consequently, some of the major goals of the medical center were to move from focusing on inpatient care to focusing on ambulatory care, from expanding hospital operations to developing alternative-care services, and from focusing on profit centers to focusing on cost centers. In its assessment of its organizational internal environment, Community Medical Center found that its hospital information system (HIS) was inadequate to support the new enterprise goals. What the medical center discovered was that the current transaction-based systems principally supported a profit-center strategy with a focus on financial systems. Patient-care tasks were only minimally supported and frequently this support was solely in operational areas such as order-entry/results reporting systems. The current system did not adequately capture or store patient-care-related data on a longitudinal basis or effectively track resource consumption. These data are precisely the type of data Community Medical Center would need in order to be a surviving player in a managed-care environment.

It is important to recognize in the Community Medical Center scenario that although Community Medical Center could develop the appropriate strategic initiatives, these initiatives were bound to fail without the appropriate information systems to support their implementation. The development of strategic information systems is critical to the success of the organization.

Levels of Organizational Decision Making

How can an information system be developed that will support organizational goals and work practices? To answer this question, a knowledge of organizational levels of decision making is necessary. Figure 2-4 is a typical representation of decision-making levels within an organization. The top level encompasses strategic decision making. It is within this purview that managers make decisions about the overall goals and direction of the enterprise. Some examples of decisions made at this level include the type of business in which the enterprise will engage (e.g., managed care), what geographical location to operate within (e.g., local, state, national), and what services to provide (e.g., acute, ambulatory, rehabilitative, long-term care). It is at this level as well that overall information technology goals should be set based on the enterprise-wide goals. Developing an integrated information architecture that supports clinical, financial, and management decision making would be an example of an information systems strategic goal. This goal would support the broader enterprise-wide goal of being a viable competitor in a managed-care environment.

The second level of decision making involves tactical decisions. It is at this level that strategies are developed that determine how organizational goals are to be achieved. Decisions at this level are made within each tactical unit. For example, marketing, patient-care services, and finance may be viewed as tactical units. From a tactical standpoint these units are concerned with implementing approaches that will achieve enterprise strate-

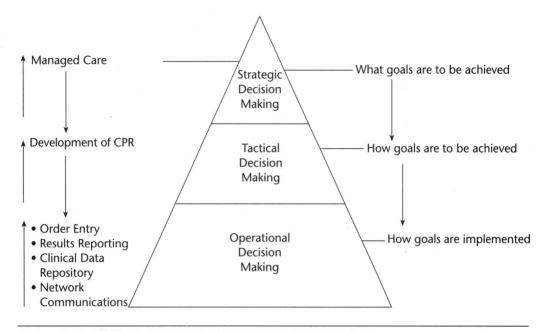

Figure 2-4. Decision-making Levels within an Organization

gic goals. The patient-care services tactical unit may determine that to achieve the goal of managed care, practice guidelines must be implemented. The unit may determine that a comprehensive, computer-based patient record (CPR) is necessary to achieve departmental goals that support the overriding organizational goal of providing managed care. The finance area may determine that departmental goals require the implementation of a sophisticated decision support system. Regardless of the decisions made at this level, they must all conform to the strategic policy of the enterprise. In the case of new information system implementation, all decisions must comply with the goal of an integrated architecture.

The third level of decision making involves the day-to-day decisions that keep the enterprise operating—how tactical decisions are implemented. This process includes hiring employees, scheduling work, ordering supplies, caring for patients, and processing patient bills.

Figure 2-5 presents a perspective of the interrelationship between the decision-making levels relative to the strategic goal of providing managed

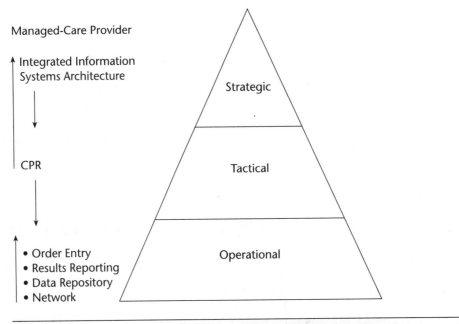

Managed-Care Provider

Integrated Information
Systems Architecture

Strategic

CPR

Tactical

• Order Entry
• Results Reporting
• Data Repository
• Network

Operational

Figure 2-5.   Interrelationships among Decision-making Levels

care and developing an integrated information systems architecture. At the strategic level, among the decisions made are goals for becoming a managed-care provider and for implementing an integrated information systems architecture. At the tactical level a decision of how these goals are to be achieved is made. In this example, one of the tactical decisions is that a longitudinal, computer-based patient record must be developed. At the operational level the computer-based patient record is implemented through an order-entry/results reporting system, a clinical data repository, clinical decision support systems, a network communications system, and so on. Thus, Figure 2-5 presents a straightforward view of the interrelationships among decision-making levels and how these might apply to an information systems example.

The Life Cycle of Information Systems in the Organization

Any study of health-care information systems has to include an examination of the life cycle of information systems within an organization. The discussion of an information system life cycle can take two perspectives. One perspective is that of the life cycle of the information system itself—that is, its development, growth, and deterioration. Another perspective is to study an organization's experience (or life cycle) with respect to information systems—that is, the **organization-wide information systems life cycle.** Both of these perspectives are very important because they clarify how organizations manage information technology and how information technologies impact the organization.

Information System Life Cycle

An information system goes through four distinct phases: development, growth, maturity, and deterioration. To be more precise in describing what occurs at each phase in the **information systems life cycle** (ISLC), labels that better identify the activities in each phase are applied. These include design (i.e., development), implementation (growth), operation and maintenance (maturity), and obsolescence (deterioration) (Martin, 1991).

At each phase in the life cycle, the activities, needs, and impact of the system are unique. A living organism will, for example, have different capabilities and needs in the development phase of its life cycle than in the maturity or deterioration phases. An infant or young child's abilities and needs, for example, are quite different from a mature adult. Similarly an information system will provide different capabilities, make different demands, and impact the organization in different ways at each stage of its life cycle.

All health-care organizations have hundreds of different information systems operating simultaneously. An organization may have administrative information systems such as MIS and DSS; clinical information systems such as a patient-care system, laboratory system, and radiology system; operational systems such as an admission/registration system, operating room scheduling system, and inventory control system; and financial systems such as billing, accounts receivable, and accounts payable. Given the number of information systems in an organization, it is easy to understand that at any one time multiple information systems will be in different phases of the life cycle. For example, the registration/admission system may be in a mature stage; the clinical laboratory system may be in the development phase; the marketing system may be in the obsolescence phase; the case-mix system may be in the design phase.

Therefore, information systems throughout an enterprise are in a constant state of fluctuation. It is highly unlikely that all information systems will be in a mature state at any given point in time. Every enterprise will constantly experience a high level of life cycle stage variability. This variability creates discontinuity, which causes stress within the organization.

The stress of discontinuity is manifested in several ways. One aspect of stress is the competition for resources. For example, the clinical laboratory may be implementing a new laboratory system. At the same time, the radiology department may be in the process of determining functionality for a new information system and the quality improvement department may be requesting enhancements to its existing system. All three systems are in different phases of the information systems life cycle. The clinical laboratory system is in the implementation phase, the radiology system is in the design phase, and the quality improvement system is in the maturity phase. Obviously, each of these systems will be competing for some of the same sets of resources at the same time, including technical assistance or people resources, hardware and software resources, financial or budgetary allocation resources, and time resources. The laboratory department will need technical assistance, training, and site preparation assistance during its implementation stage. The radiology department will need technical assistance in identifying system design. The quality improvement system will require technical expertise to perform the system upgrade and may require a greater portion of the equipment resource. All systems will bear some cost in regard to financial expenditure.

The phenomenon of discontinuity composes the usual environment in any organization and results in competition for limited resources which in turn creates organizational stress. Therefore, to lessen the organizational burden, it is important that needs are prioritized in light of organizational goals and that appropriate resources be allocated.

Information Life Cycle of the Organization

For all organizations, a composite picture of an organization-wide information systems life cycle can be visualized. Within this perspective, the experience and sophistication of organizations in managing and using information systems is studied. It would seem obvious that organizations with little experience in development, selection, and implementation of information systems would manage information resources differently than organizations with greater experience and sophistication. Specifically, an organization that is just starting to automate its information functions would have a different management emphasis of its technology than an organization where most of the information functions were automated.

✗ Nolan (1979) first described the concept of organizations having an information systems life cycle. Nolan suggests that an organization at any given point in time will be at a certain maturity or level of sophistication in deployment of information technology. He identified six stages in an organization-wide information systems life cycle: (1) initiation where the organization begins to automate information functions; (2) expansion or growth of information automation, which is usually unplanned; (3) control where the organization tries to manage information technology growth and control resources, primarily budget growth; (4) integration where the organization attempts to integrate distributed systems through organization-wide standards, policies, and procedures; (5) data administration where integrated databases are developed and information is considered a critical organization resource; and (6) maturity where growth of applications is focused on their strategic importance to the organization.

At each of these stages, the organization usually takes a different approach to management of information technology. For example, a laissez-faire attitude toward information resources management will usually occur in the early stages of initiation and expansion. In this stage the organization is likely to allow expansion of the technology with little or no organization-wide control. However, as the growth of technology expands and impacts the organization financially (i.e., significant technology expenditures), the organization tries to gain control over the resources. This is done by controlling allocation of funds for technology expansion and centralizing resources. As the organization becomes more sophisticated in its use of information technologies, it realizes the need for integration of technology and information management. In the stages of integration and data administration, the organizational emphasis is to treat information and management of its associated technologies as critical to the survival of the organization. The main focus in these stages is to distribute functions while centralizing standards for both technology and information management. In the final stage, maturity, the organization views information as a strategic resource and develops applications that further the strategic advantage of the enterprise.

It is important to be able to identify an enterprise's point in its life cycle because it helps to explain why certain policies and practices exist. For instance, if an organization is in the integration stage of the life cycle, policies and practices that impose centralized standards are likely in areas relating to network architecture, communication protocols, or productivity tools. In contrast, if an organization has only recently acquired information systems, it would be likely that there would be few policies and procedures in place that control the management of the technology. Identifying the stage of the information life cycle is important for understanding the organization's information system philosophy, practices, and culture.

Managing the Information Resource

Any discussion of information systems in the organization must include a study of how this important resource is managed. Today we live in an information society, and organizations, including health-care enterprises, recognize that information is one of their most valued commodities. Information and its associated resources must be managed just like any other important organizational resource. Health-care organizations, however, have not always valued information as an important commodity and the evolution of development of an information resource management philosophy has only recently been adopted by health-care enterprises. To understand why a new philosophy for managing information resources has only recently been embraced it is necessary to study the evolution of information systems from a general perspective.

Evolution of Information Systems

Historically, information systems within organizations were composed of manual processes or activities. The management of these manual systems was principally left to individual departments. Traditionally, each department maintained its own records, prepared its own reports, and stored its own information. The introduction of computers and their increasing use in health care during the late 1960s and 1970s witnessed some breakdown of strictly departmental systems. For example, the daily hospital census and admission/discharge list compilation was usually a function of the medical record department. The medical record department on a daily basis would collect the admission and discharge lists from the previous day from each patient-care unit. By adding the new admissions and subtracting the discharges from the previous day's census count, a current census count and roster of patients would be created. In a sense, the medical record department was in control of this information system and also was the "owner" of the information. When computerized admission and discharge systems were implemented in hospitals in the early 1970s, census calculation was no longer a departmental function. The computer and its associated databases replaced the departmental ownership of the census data. Thus, computerization made it possible for centralization of stored data files and made multiple use of data feasible.

Even with the trend toward computerization and centralization of data files, the traditional departmental philosophy toward information systems did not disappear. In the 1970s, data processing was customarily an activity that was incorporated into a functional area. The functional area usually responsible for data processing in health-care facilities was the finance department. Thus, rather than having an organization or enterprise-wide focus, data processing systems were usually directed toward the satisfying of financial information needs.

The 1980s saw the development of distinct data processing departments with a director. However, these data processing departments still reported to another manager, usually the chief financial officer (CFO). Thus, computerization of information systems during the 1970s and 1980s was focused primarily on financial and administrative systems to the neglect of other enterprise systems.

Concepts of Information Resources Management

It wasn't until the late 1980s that a new concept in the management of the information resource emerged in health care. As the health-care industry became more competitive, the need for accurate and timely information from an enterprise-wide perspective increased. This need led to the recognition that information and its associated resources had to be managed as an organizational resource. In the 1990s, the health-care industry began to embrace the concept and functions of **information resources management** (IRM) as a strategy for management of information as an organizational resource.

There are many definitions of IRM (Poppel, 1986; Barnett, 1981; Smalley, 1979), but generally the term encompasses all of the management concepts concerned with the creation, usage, storage, and eventual disposal of information in a business setting (Smalley, 1979). IRM usually provides the plan to integrate all information processes, computer and manual, and all information technologies associated with computers, telecommunications, office automation, distributed processing, and selection and implementation of computer systems. The general question answered by IRM is, "How can we coordinate and control our information activities throughout the company—automated and manual, clerical and managerial, routine and special—so that we can perform more effectively as a business?" (Smalley, 1979). The strategies used to coordinate and control the information resource usually involve (1) embracing a management philosophy that information must be managed as an organizational resource similar to capital and personnel, and (2) providing usual information services such as communications, office systems, library functions, and technology planning (Smith and Medley, 1987).

Associated with IRM concepts is the creation of a senior-level, executive position that includes oversight for all IRM functions and reporting directly to the chief executive officer of the organization. This position is usually referred to as **chief information officer** (CIO). A primary responsibility of the CIO is to set the strategic vision for information systems in the organization and to create an enterprise-wide information systems architecture including the development of organization-wide policies, standards, and procedures for information processing. The CIO of a health-care institution usually has a wide variety of responsibilities including strategic planning for information systems by integrating technology and information to meet the needs of managers, users, and customers. Other responsibilities include the allocation of resources, negotiation of hardware/software contracts, human resources management, quality improvement in information systems, and oversight of information systems operations (Johns, 1991). The departments reporting most frequently to a health-care CIO include information systems, telecommunications, management engineering, and medical records. Figure 2-6 provides a description of the management evolution of information systems in the health-care industry. This figure depicts how the focus of information systems has progressed from a narrow functional view to an enterprise-wide perspective.

Information Resources Management Organization

The previous section discussed how information systems management has generally evolved in health-care organizations. In this section, we will present an overview of how the organization of the information systems function itself has evolved. Prior to the adoption of IRM concepts, the usual

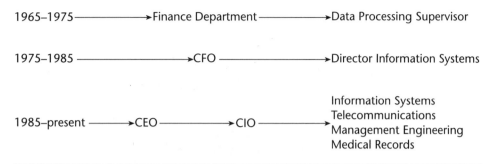

Figure 2-6. Management Organization of Information Resources

organization of the information system department was similar to that depicted in Figure 2-7. Typically the major areas included computer operations, systems, and technical support. This configuration generally coincided with the evolutionary stage the organization was in with respect to the organization information systems life cycle. It typically represented TPS and MIS systems. However, as organizations matured in their information systems life cycle, and embraced distributed systems, decision support, and end-user computing, new and different functional areas for management and operation of the information systems department

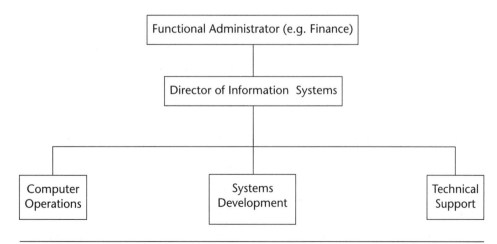

Figure 2-7. Traditional IS Department

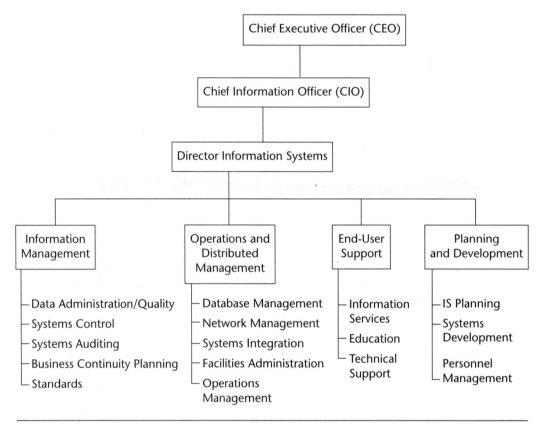

Figure 2-8.   IRM Organizational Chart

evolved. The organization that developed included more emphasis on planning functions, human resources, liaisons with other organizational areas, as well as expanded functions of traditional areas such as systems (now called development) and operations. Figure 2-8 depicts organization of the information systems department from an IRM perspective.

Impact of Information Systems Technology on the Organization

The introduction of information systems technology into the organization can have a variety of impacts. Because the influence of information technology is so great, it is often said that information systems are agents of change. Some of the impacts imposed by information systems may be positive whereas others may be viewed as negative. Because change causes stress, it is important for the health information manager to understand how the introduction of technology may change or modify the organization

Among the areas that can be affected by the introduction of information technology are job tasks, organization of social structures, employment, productivity, quality, power relationships, and organizational structures. We have already noted, through Nolan's organizational systems life cycle, how the introduction of information technology affects management practices. We have also seen how the implementation of IRM concepts can drastically alter the formal organization of an information systems department as well as the overall reporting structure of the information systems function.

In addition to these obvious impacts, the introduction of technology can also affect job tasks and employee skills. In relation to job tasks, information technology may decrease task variety and task scope. One example of a reduction of both job variety and job scope might be the introduction of technology that totally automates the process for bill generation for outpatient services. With this technology, the entire billing process from patient encounter form, to verification, to generation of the bill, may be automated. In a semiautomated environment, a billing clerk may collect patient encounter forms daily from various clinic areas. After collection of the forms, the clerk may have assigned or checked diagnostic and procedure codes on the form, verified patient insurance, and input the data into the billing program. The bill would subsequently be generated and the billing clerk might manually put the bill in an envelope for mailing.

In contrast, a totally automated process would reduce the scope and variety of tasks the billing clerk performed. In a totally automated environment, the encounter information would be entered directly by the physician or caregiver at a computer terminal. Diagnostic and procedure codes would be automatically assigned or reviewed by the computer system. Insurance verification would automatically occur through the interaction of the billing system with an insurance database. Patient demographics would be automatically checked against a patient database or clinical repository. The only task that may remain for the billing clerk might be a final verification of all information to make sure the bill is complete for processing. In this example, we can see how the introduction of technology drastically reduced both the task variety as well as task scope.

Information systems do not always decrease task variety, however. An increase of variety may be experienced when employees are relieved of repetitive and perhaps boring tasks and are allowed to focus on more challenging problems. An example is the development of a mark-sense outpatient encounter form for a specific clinic. Let's say that the medicine clinic has developed such a form containing diagnostic names and codes for the most commonly seen conditions in the clinic. The physician would complete the form by filling in a mark-sense "bubble" with a pen or pencil. For uncommon diagnoses not found on the form, the physician would write in the diagnostic name in a space provided. The form would be sent to a billing coder who would put the form through a scanner. The scanner would capture the information by the filled-in "bubbles" and transfer it to a clinical repository or database. The billing coder would manually code any uncommon diagnoses handwritten by the physician.

In this example, prior to automation of the encounter form, the billing coder had to code over and over again the common, everyday variety of diagnoses seen in the clinic. In addition, the coder had to manually enter these codes into a computer terminal. These were both repetitive and monotonous tasks. With the new system, the billing clerk is relieved of the repetitive and boring tasks and only performs the more challenging and interesting task of coding uncommon diagnoses. The reduction of task variety has actually enhanced the clerk's job.

Information systems may require that employees learn new skills. For example, the introduction of OAS requires that workers have a working knowledge of personal computers and new software tools. Information systems can also refine jobs to such an extent that a lower skill level is required after automation, for example, the total automation of the outpatient bill discussed previously. Prior to automation, the billing clerk needed to have fairly sophisticated skills in diagnostic coding. After automation, however, the billing clerk was only required to verify that all information was on the bill prior to its mailing.

Social structures and interactions can also be modified by the introduction of information technology. Information systems may either increase or decrease social interactions. Telecommunication systems such as electronic mail (e-mail) and voice mail may support additional communication and contact with people who are physically separated. Some studies have also shown that dependence on shared databases and tasks can increase interdependence and cooperation between departments (Aden, 1989). However, information technology may also physically isolate workers from the usual social interactions, such as when employees work at home.

Productivity of work may also be affected by information systems. Information systems in health care could eliminate some types of work. For example, with the development of a completely computerized patient record (CPR), the need for file clerks would be eliminated. In many cases, information systems or productivity tools have increased productivity to such an extent that positions have been eliminated. An example is in the banking industry, where 50 workers in the international money transfer department could do the work that 430 people did 10 years earlier (Lamborghini, 1982).

However, there are other studies that show there has been little displacement of workers when there has been an increase in productivity. In these cases, the same number of workers handle more work with productivity gains from increased quality of work and reduced errors (Kreamer and Danziger, 1990). A classic example in health care of the increase of productivity resulting in lower cost was the introduction of the sequential multiple analyzer computer (SMAC) in the clinical laboratory. With the introduction of this technology, the clinical laboratory was able to significantly increase the number of tests it could perform. Mount Sinai Hospital in New York performed 260,000 tests in the entire year of 1965. Once the SMAC was installed, the chemistry department was performing 8,000–10,000 tests per day with quicker results (Blum, 1986). Another example of productivity was a study whose results showed that patients in an intensive-care unit that was computerized had shorter lengths of stay with better data than those in units that were not computerized (Kjerulff, 1988).

Power relationships can also be affected by the introduction of information systems. Implementation of telecommunication systems with e-mail applications often allows workers to go outside the normal pattern of communication. Such applications make it much easier for workers to go directly to the source of information rather than through several management levels. For example, the CIO may directly e-mail a specific information systems department employee, rather than go through several management layers, to get an answer to a specific question. On the other hand, an employee may directly alert a senior management official about a situation without going through the usual communication channels.

Systems that span several departments across the organization often upset the balance of power. Since information is power, departments that closely guard or control information have significant power in the organization. As shared databases become more common in an organization, specific departmental power decreases simply because more people have more direct access to information. Likewise, the power of managers within an organization decreases as their control over information decreases. More frequently today, the direct source of information is the worker, thus increasing the power of the individual.

The Importance of Systems Thinking

In today's complex environment the need for systems thinking is imperative. Such understanding is essential for health information management professionals to perform their functions effectively. Understanding that information systems are composed of many components that must operate in support of each other and in response to an ever-changing environment is essential to the design, implementation, and operation of such systems. A large part of the job of a health information manager is problem solving, which may be in the context of how best to design an information system, how an implementation plan should be developed, or how end-users can best be trained. Each one of these examples requires an appreciation of the interdependencies among various system components. A change in one component of a system will impact another or many other system components. It is the responsibility of the health information manager to minimize adverse impact and to ensure that any system change will result in desired positive results. A fundamental understanding of systems concepts and the contribution of interrelationships between system components of people, work processes, data, information technologies, and the organization is integral to getting the job done well.

Summary

- A system is a group of flexible, self-adapting components that act through defined relationships to accomplish a goal.
- Systems can be classified in many ways. A system may be simple or complex, open or closed, stable or dynamic, permanent or temporary.

- An information system is composed of a group of component parts (people, hardware, software) that are self-adapting and that interact through defined relationships to accomplish a goal.

- Information system processes include input, process, and output with a feedback relationship between each.

- Information systems can be classified by their purpose. This classification includes transaction processing systems (TPS), management information systems (MIS), decision support systems (DSS), executive information systems (EIS), and office automation systems (OAS).

- Information systems should support various levels of organizational decision making including strategic, managerial, and operational decision levels.

- An information system has its own life cycle. The phases of the information systems life cycle (ISLC) are design, implementation, operation and maintenance, and obsolescence.

- Every organization has an organization-wide information systems life cycle. The stages of organization-wide life cycle include initiation, expansion, control, integration, data administration, and maturity.

- Information is one of the most important strategic assets of the organization. Thus, organizations have begun to embrace the concept and functions of information resources management (IRM) as a strategy for the management of information and its associated resources.

- The implementation of information systems technology into the organization introduces enormous change having a variety of impacts, both negative and positive. Thus, it is important for organizations to develop a formal program for change management.

Review Questions

1. Explain why information systems must accommodate the various levels of organizational decision making in the organization. What are the differences in these levels? What functionality must the information system have to support each of these areas?

2. Explain the differences between the information systems life cycle (ISLC) and an organization-wide life cycle. Are these two life cycles related in any way? Explain why or why not.

3. Explain the concept of discontinuity with regard to organization-wide information systems life cycle.

4. Discuss why the practices of information resources management are important for today's health-care organizations to embrace. How has the lack of adoption of these strategies affected the sophistication of information systems in health-care organizations today?

5. Discuss how implementation of information systems impact organizational culture and operations. Give some examples of how organizations can manage the change caused by adoption of information systems so that negative impact is minimized.

References

Aden, C. E. (1989). Occupational adaptation to computerized medical information systems. *Journal of Health Social Behavior, 30,* 163–179.

Alter, S. (1992). *Information systems: A management perspective.* Reading, PA: Benjamin/Cummings Publishing Co.

Barnett, A. (1981, July). Information resource management, an MIS adjunct. *Management Information Systems, 1,* 24–25.

Blum, B. I. (1986). *Clinical information systems.* New York: Springer-Verlag.

Johns, M. L. (1991). Relationship of functions performed by hospital chief information officers and organization, job, and person-related characteristics. Dissertation, The Ohio State University.

Kjerulff, K. H. (1988). The integration of hospital information systems into nursing practice: A literature review. In M. J. Ball, K. J. Hannah, U. Gerdin Gelger, and H. Peterson (eds.), *Nursing informatics.* New York: Springer-Verlag.

Kreamer, K. L., and Danziger, J. N. (1990). The impacts of computer technology on the worklife of information workers. *Social Science Computer Review, 8,* 592–613.

Lamborghini, Bruno (1982). The impact on the enterprise. In Gunter Friedrichs and Adam Schaff (eds.), *Microelectronics and society: For better or worse.* Oxford, England: Pergamon Press, pp. 119–156.

Martin, M. P. (1991). *Analysis and design of business information systems.* New York: Macmillan Publishing Co.

Nolan, R. F. (1979, March–April). Managing the crises in data processing. *Harvard Business Review*, pp. 115–126.

Poppel, H. L. (1986). *Information resource management: An overview.* Technical report 001.0001.001. Boston: Auerback Publishers.

Smalley, D. A. (1979). *Planning for information resource management.* Battelle Technical Inputs to Planning/Review No. 1, Battelle Memorial Institute, p. 4.

Smith, A. N., and Medley, D. B. (1987). *Information resource management.* Cincinnati: South-Western Publishing Co.

Chapter 3

Information Systems in Health Care

Learning Objectives

After completing this chapter, the learner should be able to:

1. Distinguish between the concepts of data, information, and knowledge and give examples of each.
2. Describe the evolution of information systems in health-care delivery.
3. Discuss how the management of information systems in health-care facilities has changed over time and how this has affected the development of information technology in health-care delivery.
4. Distinguish between in-house developed, shared, turnkey, and stand-alone information systems.
5. Provide examples of clinical and administrative information systems.
6. Discuss the elements of a hospital information system.
7. Discuss current trends in health-care information systems.

Key Terms

Administrative and Managerial Information Systems
Computer-Based Patient Record
Data

Hospital Information Systems
Information
In-house Systems
Knowledge
Laboratory Information Systems
Nursing Information Systems
Patient Monitoring Systems
Pharmacy Information Systems
Shared Systems
Stand-Alone Systems
Turnkey Systems

Introduction

Chapter 2 discusses general information systems principles and how the introduction of computers affects the organization. This chapter provides a history of information systems in health care and describes various types of information systems found in a health-care organization. It is important to reflect upon the general information systems concepts presented and try to integrate these with the discussion of health information systems that follows.

History of Information Systems in Health Care

The history of information systems in health care can be approached in a variety of ways. The evolution of information systems can be studied from the standpoint of technology, system design approaches, management approaches, or from a data–information–knowledge model. All of these viewpoints are to some extent influenced by each other. We will focus our study on the data–information–knowledge model and contrast it to the evolution of technology, system design, and management approaches.

Distinctions between Data, Information, and Knowledge

The distinction between data, information, and knowledge provides the foundation for design, development, and evaluation of information systems relative to the functions they support. Figure 3-1 shows the differences between data, information, and knowledge from a hierarchical perspective.

Data are facts, images, or sounds that may or may not be useful to a particular task. Frequently data are referred to as noninterpreted items. The number 104 is a piece of data. However, the number 104 has no meaning by itself. Depending on the context, 104 could mean anything. It could

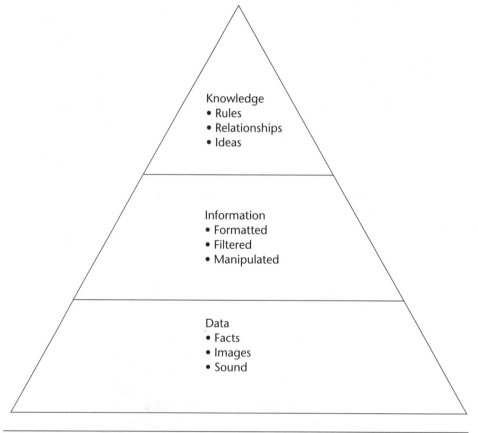

Figure 3-1.   Hierarchical View of Data–Information–Knowledge

mean an elevated temperature; it could mean a systolic pressure within normal range; it could mean tachycardia. Without a contextual reference, the number 104 has no particular meaning. Another distinguishing feature of a data system is that it processes limited amounts of data and does not maintain a long-term database. Thus, an information system can be called a data system if it only produces facts, images, or sounds without any contextual basis.

Information, on the other hand, consists of data or sets of data whose content or form is useful to a particular task. Characteristics that distinguish information systems from data systems are the maintenance of a long-term database and the use of applications built on storage, retrieval, and communication concepts (Blum, 1986). Data need to be formatted, filtered, and/or manipulated in order to be converted to information. For example, if we take the data 102, 104, 101, 100, they have no meaning. However, if we add additional data to this string of numbers and filter, format, and manipulate the data so that they read: Daily Oral Temperature of Mrs. Jones, 8/31/95: 7 A.M.: 102; 11 A.M. 104; 3 P.M. 101; 7 P.M. 100, it becomes obvious that these are four temperature readings for Mrs. Jones on August 31, 1995. Data can be converted to information in a number of ways. Data can be summarized to provide information. For instance, the data 5, 7, 3, 2, 5, 8, could be manipulated and summarized as: Average Length of Stay for the Pediatric Unit: 5 days.

Data can be highlighted to provide information. A good example is the highlighting of out-of-range or abnormal laboratory values on a computer display screen. Data can be formatted or presented in a way so as to provide information. Graphs and tables are good examples of conversions of data into meaningful information. A computer system can be termed an information system if it provides data that are formatted, manipulated, or presented in a meaningful way. Frequently, information systems are characterized as systems that "tell" us something.

Knowledge is a combination of rules, relationships, ideas, and experience. People make decisions based on current information in combination with their previous experience or knowledge of the situation. For example, the information concerning Mrs. Jones's temperature readings would be turned into knowledge by a caregiver who recognizes that the temperature readings were elevated and who combines the relationship between elevated temperature and disease processes with the information. Thus, the caregiver might surmise that the patient has an infection. Knowledge systems are usually composed of an expert knowledge base, algorithms, or some type of rule-based or decision analysis adjunct. An example of knowledge systems in the clinical area are diagnostic decision support systems (DDSS), which provide collegial assistance in making decisions to the user.

The distinctions between data, information, and knowledge sometimes become blurred and definitions or usage may vary depending on a specific discipline. From a health information management perspective, it is important to keep in mind the differences between these concepts. Ultimately these distinctions may vitally influence the design and development of a system required for specific tasks or functions.

Evolution of Information Systems in Health Care

Just like information systems in other industries, the history of information systems in health care is one of evolution. Until the late 1960s and early 1970s, information systems were largely paper based. With the development and application of information technologies in other industries, health care slowly began to adopt and modify these technologies for its own use. Figure 3-2 displays some of the key development areas.

Financial and Clinical Systems

For more than a century, information systems in health care have been paper based. These include systems for administrative, managerial, and clinical uses. Although automation has been occurring since the 1960s, the fact remains that information systems in health care, particularly in the clinical arena, still remain primarily paper based (Dick and Steen, 1991).

The initial use of computers in health care occurred during the 1960s and early 1970s. Most of these early systems focused on financial applications for several reasons. First, the implementation of automated financial systems was occurring in other industries and transfer of this technology to health care was an obvious lateral movement. Second, the nature, scope, and development of computer technology at the time supported data systems better than more sophisticated information systems. A predominant reason for the early and continued focus on financial systems related to organizational structure. As we learned previously, the data processing function usually reported to the finance department and later to the chief financial officer of the hospital. This reporting structure, in effect, restricted

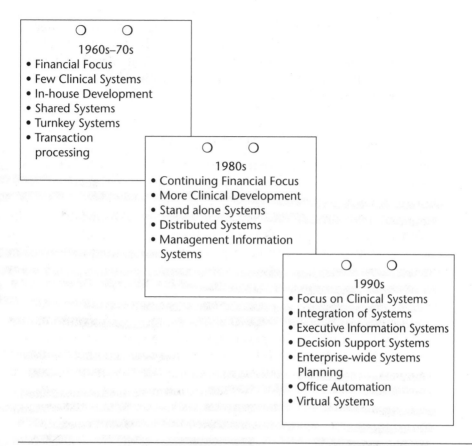

Figure 3-2. Timelining Health Information Systems Evolution

data processing applications to a specific functional area rather then facilitating an enterprisewide focus for the technology.

Although the principal focus was on automated financial systems, there were several exemplary applications in the clinical area. These included projects that focused on the development of systems for clinical information capture as well as medical decision making, for example, work associated with the MEDINET project at General Electric, the work by Bolt, Beranek, and Newsman in Cambridge, Massachusetts, and the work at Massachusetts General Hospital in Boston. A number of hospital applications were also undertaken including those by Warner at Latter Day Saints Hospital in Salt Lake City, Utah; by Collen at Kaiser Permanente in Oakland, California; by Wiederhold at Stanford University in Stanford, California; and by scientists at Lockheed in Sunnyvale, California (Blois and Shortliffe, 1990).

In-House Developed, Shared, Turnkey, and Stand-Alone Systems

The primary system alternatives in the 1960s and 1970s were either in-house developed or shared data processing services. Development of **in-house systems** included on-site systems that were designed, programmed, supported, and modified by hospital data processing staff. Usually only very large facilities such as teaching hospitals could afford the development costs associated with such projects. The advantage of the in-house development process was production of a self-styled system felt to be more flexible in meeting hospital needs than vendor-developed products. The disadvantages, however, were numerous, including high start-up costs, lengthy development process, and large technical staff requirements.

Shared data processing services were an alternative to in-house development during this period. Usually **shared systems** included those designed, programmed, and maintained by a system vendor and run on computer equipment at the vendor site. Because of the centralized nature of the system, the system and all the associated services were shared by multiple hospitals. Communication of data between hospitals and the vendor site were either through telephone lines or, in less sophisticated systems, by paper forms. The advantages of a shared services arrangement included low start-up costs, low technical staffing requirements by the hospital, and the purchase of a fully tested and proven system. Shared system arrangements are still used today, particularly by smaller hospitals. Disadvantages of a shared system include lack of system flexibility to meet specific institution needs.

Turnkey systems began to emerge in the late 1970s. Development of a turnkey system is performed by an information systems vendor. Usually development includes only the software side of the system. The turnkey system is installed on a hospital computer (frequently purchased only for that system) and operated by the hospital staff. The initial systems were called turnkey because essentially the hospital could literally just turn the system on and be ready for business. In early implementations, turnkey systems were not modifiable. What a hospital purchased is what it got.

Today, however, development tools are sometimes provided that allow hospital staff to customize the basic functions to meet hospital-specific needs. Turnkey systems were particularly attractive to smaller hospitals that desired to purchase a tested and proven system and could not afford to have a large in-house staff to either develop or modify systems. Turnkey systems usually have a fairly quick start-up with moderate start-up costs and moderate technical staffing requirements.

As automation became more sophisticated and commonplace with implementation of financial and admission/discharge systems, it also became more diversified. **Stand-alone systems** were developed to support functional tasks for separate departmental areas. With stand-alone systems, each department claimed ownership of its data. Departments maintained separate files and separate computers that supported the system. Usually there was no attempt to share information among systems. Lack of systems integration led to duplication of resources including equipment, people, and data. In addition, data that could be used on an enterprise-wide basis for decision making were difficult to provide through this decentralized approach. This disadvantage has had a lasting and significant impact on hospitals today, making it difficult to develop information and decision support systems that promote the needs of the enterprise in a managed-care environment.

Information System Types

In Chapter 2, six types of information systems are discussed: transaction processing systems (TPS), management information systems (MIS), decision support systems (DSS), executive information systems (EIS), expert systems (ES), and office automation systems (OAS). Early systems in health care were principally transaction processing systems. These systems automated operational functions such as accounting, payroll, inventory, and admission/discharge systems. Later, other transaction systems, such as order entry, were added to the capabilities. Management information systems emerged in the late 1970s and gradually became more sophisticated during the 1980s. One factor influencing the growth of MIS during this period was the introduction of the national prospective payment (diagnostic-related groups or DRGs) system for Medicare patients. Because of DRG implementation, hospitals needed information systems that provided better filtered and formatted data for making managerial and strategic decisions. The implementation of DRGs also revealed the weaknesses of current information systems in linking and integrating data. Weaknesses associated with the proliferation of stand-alone systems and the historical emphasis on financial systems became magnified during the 1980s.

The 1990s witnessed increased competition in the health-care marketplace. With the increase of health maintenance organizations (HMOs), development of alliances, and focus on managed care, a need evolved for the development of executive information and decision support systems. EIS development and implementation began to occur at the end of the 1980s. In contrast to the standardized, routine reports generated by an MIS, executive information systems are interactive systems having a user-friendly human interface that allows managers the capability of accessing information to monitor operations and business conditions. EIS became exceedingly important as managers attempted to better control operational areas and make better business decisions. Another factor that influenced the development of EIS was the beginning of building enterprisewide information architectures. These architectures focused on improvement of data communications through local, enterprise, and wide-area communication networks.

The development and implementation of optical fiber provided faster communications for both data and images. Better control over the development of enterprisewide information standards and data models has also contributed to sophisticated systems such as EIS and DSS. However, the design and implementation of an enterprisewide architecture and high-level organizational management authority over information standards is still the exception rather than the rule. With continuing external forces in the industry mandating the need for better information systems, it is expected that enterprise communication architectures will continually expand. The trend toward consolidation of, and alliances between, health-care corporations will also provide an impetus for development of such architectures and standards.

The growth of office automation (personal computers and productivity software) began in the mid-1980s. As personal computers proliferated in the late 1980s and early 1990s, opportunities arose to increase productivity. However, without an enterprisewide communication architecture and information standards, many hospitals discovered that the increase in personal computers only magnified the problem of fragmentation of information. Because many institutions still do not have an enterprisewide model for data communications or a design for interconnectivity among local-area networks (LANs), the problem of information fragmentation within health-care facilities is still significant.

Current Applications and Trends in Health-Care Information Systems

There are a plethora of information system applications in health care today. Many of these applications are clinically oriented while others support operational activities or are managerial in nature. Whatever the focus, each type of application is important in supporting the overall function of health-care delivery. While an understanding of specific systems is necessary, it is even more important for the health information manager to understand current trends that support standardization and communication of information. This section provides a view of both worlds.

Clinical Applications and Systems

Clinical or medical computing applications span a range of functions including patient monitoring, patient management systems, clinical decision support systems, and ancillary departmental systems. It is difficult to discuss exclusively any one type of system without crossing over into another system domain. For example, a nursing information system (NIS) may be defined as an ancillary system. However, components of an NIS may include patient management, decision support, and documentation functions. Therefore, the categorization and discussion of systems that follows is arbitrary with the acknowledgment that there are frequently overlaps in function and purpose among system types.

Hospital Information Systems

Broadly defined, **hospital information systems** (HIS) provide communication among health facility workers and support organizational information needs for operations, planning, patient care, and documentation. A health-care facility, such as a hospital or clinic, is an operationally complex entity. Enormous amounts of information and a high level of communication are required for optimal efficiency and effectiveness. Through communication architectures, databases, and application programs, HIS help to handle this complexity by coordinating work tasks, integrating information, organizing and storing information, and providing information for decision support.

A simple example of coordination of work tasks is the relationship between the preparation of a patient's meal and the physician's dietary order. Before a patient's meal can be prepared, the dietary department must have a physician order indicating what type of dietary regimen is appropriate. An HIS can provide for coordination between the work task of food preparation and dietary order by communicating the physician's order through an order entry system. Another example of coordination of work tasks is scheduling patients for treatment or diagnostic workup. A patient may require a visit to the radiology department for an x-ray and may also require a bedside respiratory therapy treatment. In this case, it is imperative that both radiology and respiratory therapy departments know the dates and times the patient is available for either x-ray study or therapy. An HIS can assist with this scheduling function.

As we have discussed previously, automated systems for information capture, storage, and retrieval have become essential for managerial and clinical planning and decision making. From a clinical perspective, planning can be as rudimentary as maintaining adequate inventory of drugs, supplies, instruments, and equipment. From a managerial perspective, planning can be as fundamental as determining what services should be offered, how many hospital beds should be kept in operation, and so on. An HIS can assist with these functions.

The components of an HIS will vary among institutions. No doubt, some HIS are more sophisticated than others in their functions and in the information technologies they employ. A general view of the functions that an HIS should provide has been developed by Friedman and Martin (1987). This model suggests that an HIS should be capable of performing the following functions: (1) core applications; (2) business and financial functions; (3) communications and networking; (4) departmental management; (5) medical documentation; and (6) medical support.

Centralized hospital functions such as patient scheduling, admission, and discharge are considered core applications. These applications are usually embodied in a registration–admission–discharge–transfer (RADT) system. Using a centralized database of patient demographics and history of admission, the RADT system can provide information to ancillary systems (i.e., pharmacy, radiology, laboratory, etc.), thus reducing redundancy and increasing efficiency and effectiveness.

Business and financial functions provide for the operation and management of traditional functions such as payroll, general ledger, and accounts receivable. As we have already discussed, the communications and networking systems of an HIS allow for integration of all HIS and ancillary system components. An HIS is an important "hub" for communication to systems such as pharmacy, radiology, laboratory, dietary, operating room, housekeeping, and other services. An important part of this HIS function is the order-entry–results reporting system. This system provides communication of physician orders to ancillary units and also allows ancillary units to report results of tests back to the physician and other caregivers. The mismanagement of paper orders and test results, often an enormous problem in manual systems, is reduced through this type of communication system. Departmental management systems support the internal needs of hospital departments. Among these systems are pharmacy, laboratory, radiology, and dietary information systems. Often these systems were examples of stand-alone systems that managed internal departmental functions. The results of such stand-alone systems were usually redundancy of data, differences in data definitions, and loss of efficiency from an enterprisewide perspective. In today's environment, however, the trend is to integrate, or at least interface, these systems with the core HIS applications.

Medical documentation systems perform the functions of the standard medical record in collecting, storing, and presenting clinical information. The extent of providing this function varies among HIS and to date no HIS has totally replaced the paper medical record. However, various components of the paper record have been replaced by some HIS. For example, an order-entry–results reporting capability can store the list of physician orders and results of tests, thus replacing manual order forms and test result documentation. Some HIS also include nursing system components that allow for charting of patient condition and care. Examples are medication administration records and vital signs charting. When these types of functions go beyond purely an operational focus and store data on a long-term basis, they can replace the traditional paper medical documentation systems.

Medical documentation systems can also support managerial and administrative decision making. The storage of data from these systems can provide administrators with information on trend patterns. For example, they can provide data that, when combined with financial systems, provide information about the level of efficiency of the facility in managing specific diagnoses; or the level of efficiency of specific health-care providers; or the level of effectiveness in treatment, diagnosis, and utilization of resources. Thus, when well designed and integrated with other components of the HIS, medical documentation systems can effectively support operations, management, and decision making in a number of arenas.

The final component of an HIS as proposed by Friedman and Martin (1987) constitutes support for medical decision making. Medical support systems directly assist health-care providers in interpretation of data and in making clinically related decisions. Once data from component systems (i.e., nursing, laboratory, pharmacy, etc.) are stored and integrated, these data can be used to monitor patients, issue alerts, and provide limited advice for diagnosis or therapy. A good example of such integration is drug alerts. In this case, the medication allergies of a patient might be entered through the nursing information system. When a physician orders a drug through the order entry system to pharmacy, the pharmacy system reviews the patient drug profile and allergies, checking for any contraindications. In situations where a drug has been ordered that is contraindicated or may produce an allergic reaction for a specific patient, an alert is automatically and immediately communicated to the physician. Thus, where various HIS components are integrated, higher levels of efficiency and effectiveness are likely.

Patient Monitoring Systems

Automated **patient monitoring systems** collect, store, interpret, and display physiologic patient data. Patient monitoring systems provide repeated or continuous observations or measurements of patient physiologic conditions. Patient monitoring systems were first introduced into health care in the mid- to late 1960s. Early systems were focused on narrow applications whereas today these systems frequently monitor a variety of patient physiologic parameters simultaneously. These systems provide information to clinicians and control life-sustaining devices.

Patient monitoring systems are critical in helping to detect life-threatening events. Patients who are critically ill usually have complicated therapy regimens. Because of their condition and complicated therapy, vast amounts of clinical data are accumulated. The filtering of the data becomes critical in alerting caregivers of life-threatening situations and in identifying trends and responses to therapy.

Patient monitoring systems are found in various areas of a hospital such as emergency departments, operating rooms, general acute-care units, and intensive-care units. Such systems have database capabilities as well as report generation and to some extent decision-making capabilities. Usually such systems in intensive-care units are coordinated with automated charting systems. In addition to physiologic data, they include documentation concerning medication administration, laboratory results, response to treatment, shift summaries, and so on.

Nursing Information Systems

Nursing information systems (NIS) have specific functions that support the nursing-care process both from clinical and managerial perspectives. In addition to documentation (charting) functions, NIS can help nurses in determining diagnoses, preparing and implementing of nursing-care plans, and evaluating care that was provided. NIS can support nursing management functions, such as determining the need for nursing resources, including scheduling of personnel who have the appropriate level of education, training, or skill to effectively provide care given specific situations of patient acuity and volume. NIS can also provide a valuable function in assessing quality of nursing services. More frequently this assessment is focused on the structure and process of nursing care rather than outcome.

Advancement in NIS is probably more dependent on required changes within nursing practice itself than the advancement of technology. Namely, this includes the development of taxonomies and methods for characterizing patient status, categorizing patient conditions, and creating standard patient-care plans. Before technology can be optimally applied to support nursing practice, fundamental answers must be provided to questions involving (1) the type of data required to support nursing care; (2) the nature of nursing diagnoses and objectives; (3) identification of effective nursing interventions; (4) identification of outcomes to be evaluated; and (5) identification of methods for evaluation of patient outcomes (Ozbolt, Abraham, and Schultz, 1990).

Laboratory Information Systems

Laboratory information systems (LIS) support both the processing of data associated with laboratory tests and management functions associated with day-to-day operations. Computer technology today is integrated into laboratory instruments that process specimens. The data from these analyses need to be stored, analyzed, and distributed. An LIS supports these three dimensions of information management. In addition, an LIS supports management functions such as controlling inventory, monitoring work flow, and assessing the effectiveness of the laboratory.

To understand more fully the functions of an LIS, it is important to recognize that a clinical laboratory includes many subspecialties or subareas such as clinical chemistry, hematology, clinical microbiology, cytology, surgical pathology, and blood bank. Each of these areas has its own functions to perform and has its own data processing requirements. Therefore, within an LIS, it is not uncommon to find special functions that meet the demands of each area.

The fundamental functions that an LIS performs include test ordering and results reporting, patient and specimen identification, data processing and record keeping, data acquisition, report generation, quality control, and managerial reporting (Smith and Svirbely, 1990).

Pharmacy Information Systems

Pharmacy information systems collect, store, and manage information related to drugs and the use of drugs in patient care. A primary activity of the pharmacy is to provide medications for patient care in response to a physician's order. When an order is received by the pharmacy, the pharmacist verifies it for accuracy and evaluates it against the patient's current drug therapy (i.e., what medications the patient is already taking) and clinical history. Through this process, the pharmacist is able to identify potential drug–drug interactions, contraindications with patient allergies, and/or drug sensitivities. Once the prescription is approved, the appropriate medication is retrieved from the pharmacy inventory or is formulated (made up). The order is dispensed and noted in the patient's medication profile and delivered to the nursing unit. Adjunct functions are also performed by the pharmacy to support the dispensing of drugs. These include tasks associated with inventory control, ordering of medications, providing data for billing, maintaining required records related to dispensing and administering narcotics, and developing and maintaining the hospital or clinic formulary.

Functions supported by a pharmacy information system include online order entry, pharmacist review, medication profile update, label printing, drug-dispensing reports, medication administration reports, inventory maintenance and automatic drug reorder, drug-use reports, and controlled-drug reports (Speedie and McKay, 1990). In addition to providing information management internal to the pharmacy, many pharmacy information systems support business functions such as generating bills and collecting information on pharmacy department productivity, sales volume, prescription activity, and drug usage.

Other Clinically Oriented Information Systems

The previous discussion presents a few examples of the types of clinically oriented information systems that may exist in a health-care facility. Certainly the breadth and depth of applications for information management literally reach out to every area within a health-care organization. For example, common clinically oriented systems include radiology information systems (RIS), dietary information systems, emergency department systems, as well as support systems for central supply, operating room systems, anesthesia systems, and so on. A comprehensive discussion of clinical systems can be found in the text by Shortliffe and colleagues (1990).

It is not important that health information managers know the details of every clinically oriented system. Rather, the important concept is to recognize that, no matter where the information technology is applied, it must first and foremost support the tasks and information needs of the user in such a way that the information functions do not detract from or interfere with the normal work flow.

Administrative and Management Applications

Administrative and management applications, particularly in the financial area, were the first functions that were widely deployed in health-care facilities. As we discussed previously, there were many reasons responsible for this development including the reporting structure of data processing departments, previous experience in other industries with financial systems, and the focus of developing systems on a financial rather than patient-oriented approach. Frequently, however, when they coexisted in the same facility, clinical and financial systems rarely interfaced or were integrated.

In addition to poor integration between clinical and financial systems, there often exists poor integration among various managerial and administrative systems. The adverse impact of this situation has become more and more evident as competition in the health-care industry grows and as hospitals and other health-care organizations find that they do not have appropriate integration of information for decision making. Thus, when examining any health-care application, whether clinical or managerial in nature, an important question to ask is, "To what extent should this system interface with other enterprise systems?"

Financial Information Systems

Health-care organizations since the mid-1960s have recognized the opportunity for efficiency through automation of financial systems. Initially these systems automated accounting functions such as payroll preparation, accounts payable, patient accounting (billing and accounts receivable), general ledger, and budgeting. With the implementation of DRGs in the early 1980s, the need for case-mix management systems and integration of clinical and financial systems was recognized. In the managed-care environment, the emphasis on cost accounting systems and case-mix management is even greater along with decision support systems that take advantage of integrated data repositories.

Human Resource Management Information Systems

Human resource management information systems have traditionally automated functions such as maintaining and updating employee records. These systems have, however, grown in sophistication with the recognition that automation can improve efficiency. With an excess of 60 percent of a hospital's operating budget going toward employee payroll and benefits, it is important for organizations to have access to data for monitoring productivity, assessing personnel-related barriers to productivity, and determining appropriate levels of human resources mix. Today, human resource systems usually include functions for capture, storage, and manipulation of personnel data. Capabilities and display tools for various analysis are also usually incorporated, including analyzing labor reports by cost center, monitoring turnover and absenteeism, and producing productivity and quality-control analyses.

Materials Management Systems

The management of inventory and purchasing of materials and supplies is an enormous challenge to any health-care organization. Without automated systems for materials management, it would be difficult to efficiently operate a health-care organization. Materials management systems usually encompass front-end processes, such as handling requisitions for supplies and materials from departments, and back-end processes, such as managing inventory and ordering materials and supplies. A study conducted by Sneider and Murphy (1987) found that such systems provided significant benefits. Among these were reductions in inventory, improvements in bid and contracting procedures, updating of daily patient charges, improvements in avoiding lost patient charges, interface with accounts payable to obtain payment discounts, and reductions in labor costs.

Facilities Management Information Systems

Facilities are considered one of the most critical resources within an organization. Well-maintained physical facilities are essential for the provision of quality patient care as well as providing a pleasing atmosphere for workers and patients and their families. Facilities management information systems include the capture, storage, and manipulation of data used to monitor preventive maintenance, energy management, and project (construction) scheduling. Several studies have concluded that the use of such systems helps in organizational efficiency. Sedor (1989), for example, found that the potential benefits of automated facility maintenance systems included cost savings through reduced inventory of spare parts, reduced staffing of housekeeping and maintenance personnel through improved scheduling, and improved risk management.

Strategic Planning, Quality Improvement, and Decision Support

Since the late 1980s, hospitals have gradually been adopting automated systems to aid in strategic decision making, quality improvement, and decision support. The attributes of DSS and EIS are discussed earlier in the chapter. Information, both external and internal to the organization, is necessary for good strategic decision making. From an external perspective, a health-care enterprise must understand the environmental context, know the strength and weaknesses of its competition, and understand opportunities upon which it can capitalize. From an internal perspective, the enterprise must recognize its own internal strengths and weaknesses and how these can be enhanced or minimized. Thus, information systems for strategic decision making must integrate data from internal as well as external databases. The type of strategy employed by the enterprise in regard to strategic decision making will often impact the type of system and/or data required.

DSS complement systems that provide information for strategic decision making by supplying tools for the manipulation of data and presenting answers to what-if scenarios. Common DSS in health care today include forecasting systems, marketing systems, cost-accounting systems, and case-mix systems. DSS are becoming increasingly important as enterprises enter alliances with each other or enter into managed-care contracts. The survival of an enterprise in tomorrow's world will be directly related to how good decisions were made today. A fundamental component to good decision making is good information.

Automation is increasingly being used in assessment of quality of care. Quality improvement systems in clinical areas frequently focus on utilization management activities, critical path or practice guideline implementation, monitoring of critical indicators, assessment of severity of illness in comparison to patient outcomes, and case-mix analysis. As more and more attention is focused on quality at a reasonable cost, health-care organizations will be required to provide the type of data generated from such systems.

Current Trends in Health Information Systems

Current trends in health-care information systems can be viewed from several different perspectives. For example, systems can be examined in relation to trends in management of the resource, architecture, applications, communications, and technology. The health information manager must recognize that information technology is volatile—that is, what is current today is almost immediately outdated tomorrow. Therefore, any reference to specific technologies becomes unimportant. More important is a general assessment of where the information systems road is leading and how current technologies can be best incorporated to help navigate the information highways of the future and strategically position the health-care enterprise. Today's vision must be toward fully integrated systems supported by flexible data models, communication technologies, and tools that enhance decision making, improve quality and productivity, and reduce administrative costs.

Clinical Information Systems

Certainly in the 1990s a predominant emphasis is on the design, development, and implementation of a computer-based patient record (CPR). With the publishing of the seminal work on the CPR (Dick and Steen, 1991), the Institutes of Medicine (IOM) pushed to the forefront the recognized need for a longitudinal, computer-based patient record. The CPR has been defined by the IOM report as an "electronic patient record that resides in a system specifically designed to support users by providing accessibility to complete and accurate data, alerts, reminders, clinical decision support systems, links to medical knowledge, and other aids" (Dick and Steen, 1991).

The benefits of a CPR cited by the report include improvement in support and quality of patient care, enhanced productivity and reduction of administrative costs, and improved support for clinical and health services research. There have been attempts in the past to automate the patient record with varying degrees of success. It should be noted that the IOM report states that there are no demonstrations or implementations of a completely automated patient medical record. Even with the limited success of previous attempts at automation, the IOM committee that prepared the report feels that the time is right for reinitiation of this effort. The committee cites five environmental conditions that make the 1990s a right time to pursue a CPR. These conditions are (1) increase of demands for patient-related data; (2) availability of technologies that can support development and implementation of a CPR; (3) more widespread use of automation generally in society; (4) increase of volume of information needed to be managed due to a more mobile and aged population; and (5) pressures for health-care reform that require evaluation, consolidation of data, and improved communication.

The CPR will require a number of technologies including the development of clinical data repositories; application of communication technologies to link various repositories, information sources, and users; development of enterprisewide and interenterprise data models; application of technologies such as voice entry to improve user input; development of artificial intelligence and decision support systems; development of communications and other standards; integration of voice, text, data, and image processing systems; and development of policies, procedures, and methods that will ensure security of patient-related data and communications.

Administrative Information Systems

Administrative and managerial information systems in the mid-1990s and beyond will focus on the development of systems that support strategic management and decision making, and increase communications both intra- and extraorganizationally. E-mail will be used to improve and distribute communication and information. The emphasis will be on fully integrated systems that provide timely, accurate, and complete information to decision makers and knowledge workers at every level of the organization. These systems will require integration of voice, text, data, and in some instances image processing systems. Better and more sophisticated user-interface development will be required including the use of voice systems for input and query. Executive workstation design will be a focus with the development of improved methods for data inquiry. Improved systems for decision support and analysis, particularly in areas related to cost accounting, case-mix management, quality management, and productivity, will be required.

Management of the Information Resource and Standards Development

As the importance of information is recognized at top enterprise levels, the organization for management of the information resource will become more sophisticated. A distinction between information technology and systems and information management will emerge. The result will be an expanded role for information resources management at a top organizational level position reporting directly to the chief executive officer. This top-level executive (CIO) will provide vision and leadership for the organization in the strategic planning, implementation, and operation of enterprisewide information systems. In addition, this person will play a vital role on the leadership team in helping to define the strategic objectives of the organization as a whole. The information management function will become an enterprisewide objective and its direction finally disembodied from "a" functional area. Health-care organizations will finally evolve into Nolan's later stages of the information systems life cycle.

In addition to changes in organizational structure, the mid-1990s and beyond will see increased emphasis on standards development for health-care information interchange. Many types of standards are required for information interchange including: formatting and protocols; exchange standards for system interfaces; nomenclature standards for uniform vocabulary use; and consensus standards for authentication of electronic medical records (Wakerly, 1994). Many groups are involved in establishing such standards, such as the American National Standards Institute (ANSI), the American College of Radiologists/National Electrical Manufacturers Association/Digital Imaging Communications Group (ACT/NEA/DICOT), the American Society for Testing and Materials (ASTM) and the Health Level Seven (HL7). In 1994, the CPR Institute identified acceleration of standards development as a top priority. With the development and adoption of such standards, communication links among databases and other information sources will become much more feasible.

The Virtual Health-Care Information System

Development of the CPR, use of internal and external information sources by organization workers, and use of internal information sources by individuals outside the organization will all influence the development of a virtual information system. In a virtual information system, health-care enterprises must view their information resource from the perspective of virtual reality—that is, the view of information must go beyond the perspective of an information system confined to the boundaries of an organization. Rather the view must be expanded outward from the organization. Critical data no longer reside exclusively within the confines of the organization and its data bank. In effect, critical data can reside anywhere, either internal or external to the organization. Thus, the information resource becomes a virtual resource no longer residing in one place, in one format, or accessed locally. With the development and implementation of physician–health-care-facility communication links, third-party–health-care-facility communication links, government–health-care-facility communication links, alliance and partner–health-care-facility communication links, and customer/client–health-care-facility communication links, the concept of virtual information systems must be embraced if a health-care enterprise is to survive.

Summary

- The initial use of computers in health-care information processing occurred during the 1960s and early 1970s. Most of these early systems focused on financial applications. During the mid-1980s and early

1990s, a more concentrated interest focused on the development of clinical information systems.

- The primary system alternatives in the 1960s and 1970s were in-house developed or shared systems. Turnkey systems began to emerge in the late 1970s. Frequently these systems served one functional purpose and did not integrate with other organizational systems.

- The distinction between data, information, and knowledge is important. Data are facts, images, or sounds. Information consists of data or sets of data whose content or form is useful to a particular task. Knowledge is a combination of rules, relationships, ideas, and experience.

- Clinical applications and systems in health care include hospital information systems (HIS), patient monitoring systems, nursing information systems (NIS), laboratory information systems (LIS), pharmacy information systems, and other clinically related systems.

- Among administrative and management applications are financial information systems; human resources management information systems; materials management systems; facilities management information systems; and strategic planning, quality improvement, and decision support systems.

- In the 1990s and beyond, a predominant emphasis in health-care information systems will be the design and development of a computer-based patient record (CPR). The CPR is an electronic patient record that resides in a system specifically designed to support users by providing accessibility to complete and accurate data, alerts, reminders, clinical decision support systems, links to medical knowledge, and other aids.

Review Questions

1. Distinguish between data, information, and knowledge, providing examples of each.

2. Discuss the evolution of information systems in health care and explain the reasons why the early focus was on financial information system development.

3. Name and describe the functions of the following clinical information systems: hospital information system, nursing information system, patient monitoring system, laboratory information system, and pharmacy information system.

4. Name and describe the functions of the following administrative information systems: financial information system; human resource management information system; materials management system; facilities management system; and strategic planning, quality improvement, and decision support systems.

5. Discuss some of the current trends in the development and application of clinical and administrative information systems.

Enrichment Activities

1. Visit a local health-care enterprise in your area. Schedule an interview with the chief information officer and the director of the health information management department to discuss the evolution of health information systems over the past decade and the directions of information systems in the next 5 years. Discuss how the organization has adapted to the impact of change brought about by increased information systems implementation. How has this change been handled by the organization? In what stage of the organization-wide life cycle is the organization currently?

2. Tour the information systems and the health information management departments of a local health-care enterprise and observe the functional capabilities of one or more clinical information systems.

References

Blois, M. S., and Shortliffe, E. H. (1990). The computer meets medicine: Emergence of a discipline. In E. H. Shortliffe, L. E. Perreault, G. Wiederhold, and L. M. Fagan (eds.), *Medical informatics: Computer applications in health care*. Reading, MA: Addison-Wesley Publishing Co.

Blum, B. I. (1986). *Clinical information systems.* New York: Springer-Verlag.

Dick, R. S., and Steen, E. B. (1991). *The computer-based patient record: An essential technology for health care.* Washington, DC: National Academy Press.

Friedman, B. A., and Martin, J. B. (1987). Hospital information systems: The physician's role. *Journal of the American Medical Association, 257,* 1792.

Ozbolt, J., Abraham, I. L., and Schultz II, S. (1990). Nursing information systems. In E. H. Shortliffe, L. E. Perreault, G. Wiederhold, and L. M. Fagan (eds.), *Medical informatics: Computer applications in health care.* Reading, MA: Addison-Wesley Publishing Co.

Sedor, P. (1989, May 20). Automated maintenance. *Hospitals,* pp. 72–73.

Shortliffe, E. H., Perreault, L. E., Wiederhold, G., and Fagan, L. M. (eds.). (1990). *Medical informatics: Computer applications in health care.* Reading, MA: Addison-Wesley Publishing Co.

Smith, J. W., Jr., and Svirbely, J. R. (1990). Laboratory information systems. In E. H. Shortliffe, L. E. Perreault, G. Wiederhold, and L. M. Fagan (eds.), *Medical informatics: Computer applications in health care.* Reading, MA: Addison-Wesley Publishing Co.

Sneider, R. M., and Murphy, J. F. (1987, February). Automated material management systems. *Hospital Material Management Quarterly,* pp. 40–47.

Speedie, S. M., and McKay, A. B. (1990). Pharmacy systems. In E. H. Shortliffe, L. E. Perrault, G. Wiederhold, and L. M. Fagan (eds.), *Medical informatics: Computer applications in health care.* Reading, MA: Addison-Wesley Publishing Co.

Wakerly, R. T., ed. (1994). *Community health information networks.* Chicago: American Hospital Association.

Chapter 4

Strategic Planning for Information Systems

Learning Objectives

After completing this chapter, the learner should be able to:

1. Discuss the importance of linking the development of information systems to the strategic business objectives of the organization.
2. Discuss the components of business strategic planning.
3. Discuss factors that are critical to the success of the business strategic planning process.
4. Discuss various methods for information systems strategic planning.
5. Identify strengths and weaknesses of various information systems planning methods.
6. Identify critical components of an information systems strategic planning process.
7. Given an information systems strategic plan, critique its strengths and weaknesses.

Key Terms

Critical Success Factors
Environmental Analysis
Gap Analysis
Internal Analysis
Strategic Planning
SWOT Analysis

Introduction

Information engineering is one of the primary domains of practice of the health information manager. As presented in Chapter 1, this domain includes tasks associated with planning, analysis, design, and development of information systems on an enterprise-wide basis. Specifically, as depicted in Figure 4-1, these tasks include strategic planning, data modeling, process modeling, data administration, and screen and report design.

The design of enterprise information systems should be tied to the strategic planning efforts of the organization. Strategic planning for the organization involves identifying the goals and critical success factors of the enterprise. In Chapter 2, the concept of linking the development and deployment of information systems to business strategic objectives is presented in a scenario for Community Medical Center. Revisiting this scenario presents a foundation for the concepts discussed later in this chapter.

In 1993, Community Medical Center developed a strategic plan for the enterprise that focused on developing strategies to become a viable player in a capitation environment. Community Medical Center recognized that because of several external forces, it had to change its organizational structure and work practices away from a fee-for-service environment. Consequently, some of the major goals of the medical center were to move from focusing on inpatient care to focusing on ambulatory care, from expanding hospital operations to developing alternative-care services, and from focusing on profit centers to focusing on cost centers. In its assessment of its organizational internal environment, Community Medical Center found that its hospital information system (HIS) was inadequate to support the new enterprise goals. What the Medical Center discovered was that the current transaction-based systems principally supported a profit-center strategy with a focus on financial systems. Patient-care tasks were only minimally supported and frequently this support was solely in operational areas such as order-entry/results reporting systems. The current system did not adequately capture or store patient-care-related data on a longitudinal basis or effectively track resource consumption. These data are precisely the type of data Community Medical Center would need in order to be a surviving player in a managed-care environment.

This scenario effectively demonstrates that in order for any organization to be successful and competitive, its information resources must sup-

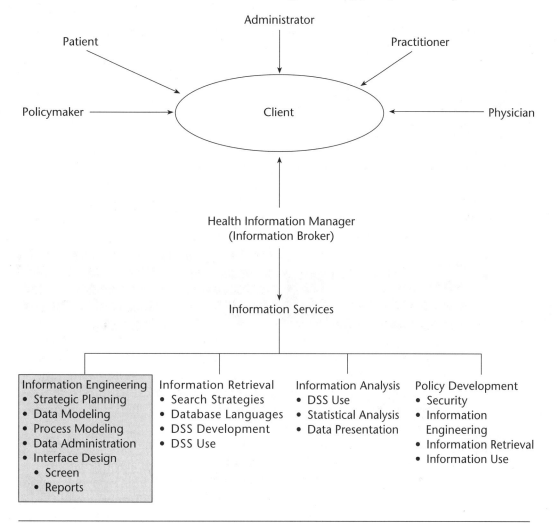

Figure 4-1.   Information Engineering Function

port critical functions and strategic objectives. Thus, the planning for information systems must be based on knowledge of the health-care organization and its critical goals or success factors. Often the "goodness" of an information system is measured by its effectiveness and its efficiency. However, the true measure of success of any information system is how well it supports the strategic initiatives of the organization or provides a competitive advantage for the enterprise. The following sections of the chapter explore general concepts related to organizational strategic planning and how the results of this process are used to strategically plan for information systems.

Health-Care Organizational Strategic Planning Process

Since the 1950s, techniques and processes for business planning have continuously evolved and have become more sophisticated. Because of the continuing competitive nature of the health-care environment since the 1980s, health-care organizations increasingly have adopted **strategic planning** processes. Although the particular methods of strategic business planning processes may vary, planning for strategic positioning of the organization usually includes four areas of focus: (1) assessing the enterprise's competitive position; (2) determining ways or alternatives for the enterprise to move ahead; (3) assessing the feasibility of various alternatives; and (4) selecting alternatives and implementing them (Boar, 1993; Ward, Griffiths, and Whitmore, 1990). The culmination of the business strategic planning process results in the development of a plan that sets the direction of the organization. Specifically this will result in a document that states the vision and mission of the enterprise and includes organizational goals, tactics, and actions that must be accomplished for the organization to maintain a competitive position.

Depending on the size and complexity of the organization, the business planning process may take from 6 to 12 months to complete. To be successful, the planning process must include several individuals to assist in data gathering and various analyses and assessments. In addition to human resources, conducting a successful planning process also requires other resources such as equipment, clerical assistance, and space. Thus, the first step in business strategic planning is the organization of resources to support the process.

Organizing Resources

For any strategic planning to be successful, there must be top management support. The commitment and visible involvement of senior management in strategic planning sends a message of resolve to the entire organization. Fundamentally this support says that strategic planning is essential to the survival of the organization.

The Planning Team

Usually top management support is represented by the establishment of a planning team consisting of the senior administrative officials in the organization. Minimally these should include the chief executive officer (CEO), chief operating officer (COO), chief financial officer (CFO), and chief information officer (CIO) and the senior vice presidents or executives of the various organizational function areas. In some cases, other organization stakeholders may be included in the planning team. These individuals may include other organization employees, customers (i.e., physicians, patients), suppliers, or community members. Ideally the planning team should consist of no more than twelve individuals. Too small a team may restrict the number of viewpoints or dimensions that should be included in brainstorming ideas, performing analyses, and analyzing and selecting alternatives. Too many individuals on the team will make coordination difficult.

Hiring a Facilitator

Frequently organizations will hire an outside consultant to facilitate the planning process. There are several reasons why an organization would want to employ a facilitator. An individual outside the organization who coordinates the planning process may be perceived to be a neutral participant. A perception of neutrality is important. If planning team members or organization employees perceive that the entire planning process was biased from the start, buy-in to the resulting plan and support for goals and action plans will be difficult to achieve.

An outside consultant may also be hired because the organization does not feel that it has the internal expertise to coordinate the planning process. Outside facilitators or consulting firms have usually conducted many strategic planning efforts. Their experience in coordinating planning activities, running meetings, bringing groups to consensus, and conducting analyses can make the planning process run significantly smoother than if an internal individual with lesser experience were to coordinate activities. Additionally, consulting companies can draw on the variety of expertise within their firms. For example, a consulting firm may have experts in meeting facilitation, change management, implementation, and evaluation.

In addition to these benefits, outside consultants can usually bring a "big picture" to the planning process. Because of their experience, consultants may have a broad perspective of the environmental factors that may positively or negatively affect the enterprise. They may have specific insights about direct competitors. Since consultants frequently work across industries, their experiences outside of health care with other businesses may provide useful perspectives.

Other Resources

Many resources are needed during the process of strategic planning. Sufficient clerical support is an absolute necessity. The planning team and its associated task forces will need to conduct exhaustive searches for information. This means accessing various information sources and databases. Information must be filed, stored, categorized, and analyzed. In addition, minutes of meetings and other documentation of planning activities must be maintained. Some organizations will use the services of information brokers or librarians to assist in the process.

Office equipment to support the process will be needed, including office furniture, computers, printers, and other tools. Space for the facilitator and clerical support staff to work is also needed as well as conference room space for planning team members and task forces to meet.

Development of Task Groups

The business strategic planning effort is much too complex for the planning team to perform alone. Usually several task groups are formed to help with the planning process. These task forces usually perform much of the "legwork" for the planning team. At a minimum, usually two task groups are formed: one task force to perform an external or environmental analysis and another to perform an internal analysis of the organization. The makeup of team members varies. Usually members of either team are employees who have diverse backgrounds, knowledge of the organization, and knowledge of the industry.

Environmental and Internal Analyses

After a planning team has been selected, task forces formed, and resources organized, the first steps in the planning process are to conduct an external or **environmental analysis** and an internal analysis of the organization. The results of these analyses will provide the underpinning for the entire strategic business plan. Therefore, it is important that these analyses be thoughtfully and carefully conducted. The purpose of the external analysis is to provide information about factors outside the organization that may positively or negatively affect the enterprise's competitive position. The purpose of the internal analysis is to learn about the organization, how it functions, and what factors are critical to its success. Ideally the analyses should be conducted concurrently so that results are available together for the planning team to review.

Environmental Analysis

It only makes sense that the environment in which a health-care organization exists has an impact on many facets of the organization. Changes in the economy, demographics, politics, legislation, or other factors in the environment will directly determine opportunities and threats for the organization. In order to maximize opportunities and minimize threats, the health-care organization must have an excellent understanding of and appreciation for the environment in which it exists. Take, for example, Anycity, USA. In Anycity, the majority of workers are employed by one aerospace company. This aerospace company provides health insurance for all of its 4,000 employees and their families, which amounts to health-care coverage for about 12,000 individuals. If for any reason this company has economic problems and is forced to cut back on its labor force, the number of individuals covered by health insurance in the community will be reduced. The economic problems of this company will trickle throughout the community. The reduction of covered individuals will directly impact health-care organizations within the community. Most likely there will be a reduction in utilization of elective health-care services, such as office visits, elective treatments, elective surgeries, and so on. This cutback, of course, will have a negative economic impact on the health-care organizations in the community.

Because changes in the external environment can significantly affect the well-being of an organization, a careful assessment of these forces is essential. Therefore, information is collected about national (and perhaps even international) political, economic, social, legal, and technological environmental forces. The task force will collect documents, read papers from think-tanks, survey journals, newspapers, and magazines, and search databases. Often, external experts will be brought together by the organization for panel presentations on specific issues. As previously mentioned, librarians or information brokers may be hired to search for and collect data from a number of electronic databases or other information sources.

In addition to scanning the national environment to identify trends, threats, and opportunities, the external analysis usually includes an assessment of the health-care industry specifically as well as an analysis of the organization's direct competitors. Understanding the forces of change within the health-care industry is absolutely essential to successful planning. These are the forces that should be actively monitored by the organization. The organization usually has a better opportunity to influence industry-specific forces than national or international forces. The internal analysis task force will use similar data-gathering techniques as those used for the external analysis. They may augment literature searching and scanning of journals and newspapers with networking within the industry. This may include attending conferences, joining professional organizations, and meeting with others in the field. In addition, information about pressure groups and stakeholders specific to the health-care industry will be gathered.

Knowledge of the organization's direct competitors is equally important. Knowing about a competitor's customer base, financial position, productivity, services, and critical success factors can provide useful information in competitively positioning an organization.

Internal Analysis

The **internal analysis** is conducted to gain an understanding about the way the organization functions. Frequently, senior management and others have imperfect views of the way the organization operates. The goal of the internal analysis is to develop a factual portrait of the organization. Data gathering for the internal analysis usually consists of reviewing various organizational documents, interviewing senior management and others, and conducting surveys.

One of the most significant outcomes of an internal analysis is identifying organizational **critical success factors**. Critical success factors (CSF) are the "limited number of areas in which results, if they are satisfactory, will ensure successful competitive performance for a business. They are the few key areas where 'things must go right' for the business to flourish" (Rockart, 1979). CSFs are important factors that help executives and the organization achieve their goals. For example, one goal of a health-care enterprise may be to increase its market share by 10 percent. Critical success factors to achieve this goal may include (1) competitive pricing, (2) local advertising, and (3) the location of care centers in strategic locations.

CSFs are usually identified through an interview process. Members of the internal task force interview senior management to determine the organizational CSFs. Managers at the director level are also interviewed to determine the CSFs for individual functional areas. Figure 4-2 graphically depicts the interrelationships between organizational, business unit, and manager CSFs.

In relation to information systems planning, CSFs should provide the guiding direction for development of systems, applications, and the use of information technology. For example, if competitive pricing is one of the most important areas for things to go right, then an information system needs to be developed that will provide senior management with the data they need to set competitive prices. This may mean the development of an information system that links to outside information sources, external data banks, and internal data banks, and provides for modeling and decision support.

Bringing the External and Internal Analyses Together

Results of the internal and external analyses are usually reported in a summary document. The purpose of this document is not so much to summarize the findings of each analysis but to emphasize areas of agreement and disagreement and to identify goals, CSFs, strengths and weaknesses, and provide an assessment of implications of trends for future direction and success of the organization. To produce this summary document, the task forces charged with the internal and external analyses usually work together to review results, trends, and assumptions.

Various tools and techniques are used to compare and analyze the results of the internal and external analyses. Among these are gap, situational, driving force, competitive forces, and value chain analyses. A **gap analysis** is a structured analysis that results in the identification of discrepancies between the way the organization sees itself and its true position vis-à-vis its competitors and other driving forces in the external environment. For example, perhaps the results of the external analysis suggest that middle-income, health-insured individuals receive more of their information about services and commodities from newspapers than from radio advertisement. In contrast, an underlying assumption by health-care senior management is that it could increase market share through more radio advertisement. If this discrepancy between the impact of newspaper versus radio advertisement was not identified, the health-

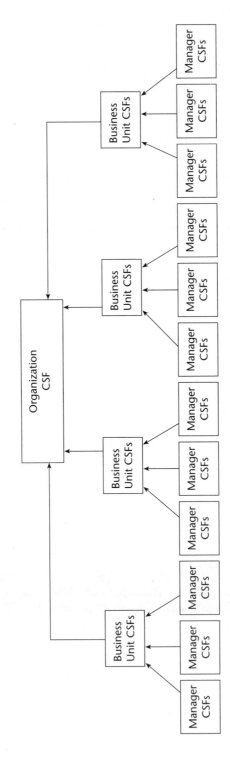

Figure 4-2. Relationship among Business Unit and Organizational Critical Success Factors

care organization could spend enormous amounts of money on a marketing plan that was destined for failure.

A frequently used technique to assess results of the internal and external analyses is the situational or **SWOT** (strengths, weaknesses, opportunities, and threats) **analysis.** This technique helps the organization assess its current position in relation to the competitive market. Strengths, weaknesses, opportunities, and threats are usually assessed by each critical success factor and also by each functional area. To illustrate how the SWOT analysis might be used, let's take an example of a large university hospital that must transition itself to meet the market demands for managed care. Let's assume that this hospital has identified several CSFs to make it competitive: (1) provide comprehensive range of clinical services, (2) maintain a strong financial position, and (3) maintain efficient operations. A SWOT analysis would evaluate each of these CSFs to determine the hospital's strengths, weaknesses, opportunities, and threats. Table 4-1 shows how such an analysis might look.

Table 4-1 is just one example of how an organization can begin to assess how it stands in relation to obtaining the CSFs that it feels are crucial to its success. A SWOT analysis can also be performed by functional area for each CSF. For example, Table 4-2 shows how a matrix could be developed to assess the CSF of efficient operations by three organizational departments. Doing a situational analysis by CSF and by functional area will give the planning team insight into the competitive position of the organization. Additionally, information from the SWOT analysis can be used in brainstorming to help the planning team determine ways to capitalize on the organization's strengths and exploit opportunities while minimizing weaknesses and threats.

Other types of analyses that are performed include driving force, competitive forces, and value chain analyses. A driving force analysis concentrates on how best to optimize the one most important focus of the business. Another technique that can be used is a competitive force analysis. This framework was originally developed by Michael Porter (1980). It focuses on the organization's critical success factors in relation to new entrants to the marketplace, substitute products or services, customers, and suppliers. If the planning team discovers that most of the organization's CSFs are associated with only one area (e.g., new entrants to the marketplace), then the team knows that the organization is neglecting to look at threats and opportunities in other areas that are important for competitive position.

Table 4-1.   SWOT Analysis by CSF

Critical Success Factors	Range of Clinical Services	Financial Position	Efficient Operations
Strengths	Patient/family-centered system of care delivery	Strong patient-care revenues	Patient-centered approach to care
	Range of outpatient and nonacute services including clinics, hospice, and long-term care	Strong collection of receivables	Critical paths operational Low length of stay Good patient-care outcomes
Weaknesses	No home health program	Large portion of uncompensated care	Information system architecture
	No cost-accounting system for patient services	No cash capital plan	Weak technology management practices
	Costs are noncompetitive in local area		No cost accounting
Opportunities	Develop longitudinal patient-care delivery process	Increase non-patient-care revenues	Publicize model programs
	Increase national and international referrals	Enhance fund-raising activities	
Threats	Other major health enterprises may be more cost competitive	Increase in uncompensated care	Managed care advancing into local area sooner than anticipated

The value chain analysis is another technique often used with information gathered from the internal analysis. This technique is discussed at length by Porter (1985). The value chain is a way of looking at the contribution of various primary and secondary functions of a business unit to the development of a product. Each function associated with production of a product adds value as well as cost to the final product. This process

Table 4-2.   SWOT Analysis by Functional Area and Efficient Operation CSF

	Information Systems	*Business Office*	*Emergency Department*
Strengths			
Weaknesses			
Opportunities			
Threats			

can alert the planning team to the most critical functions of the enter-prise—those functions that add the most value to the products.

Summary Paper Preparation

After all information from the internal and external analyses is studied, a summary paper is prepared. The purpose of this paper is to focus on the strengths, weaknesses, and opportunities for the enterprise. The paper should include a discussion of goals and critical success factors and how these compare with direct competitors. The paper should lay the founda-tion for generating options and actions by discussing implications of trends for the future and how these relate to the success of the enterprise. The summary paper should provide a realistic appraisal of the true state of the organization.

Generating Options and Developing an Enterprise Strategy

After the summary paper is studied, it is the planning team's responsibil-ity to generate options and develop an enterprise strategy for the organi-zation. The planning team should generate a small number of options for the organization to pursue and evaluate these options in terms of required resources, costs, risks, and value. These options should be linked to the goals and critical success factors previously identified through the internal and external analyses. As an example, say that a goal of Community Hos-pital and Health Care is to increase its market share in outpatient care. One option that may be pursued is to establish family practice clinics in several suburban areas of the community. Another option may be to pursue an aggressive marketing program that includes referral and hot lines for medical information, free wellness checks or screenings at area shopping malls, or a free newsletter that will reach a significant part of the market. Another option may be a program for more aggressive contract marketing to managed-care organizations.

The final part of strategic planning is the development of the enterprise strategy itself. All elements of the process are brought together and organized in a plan for action. This encompasses development or refinement of the organizational vision, mission statement, and goals. It also means that the primary goals of the organization are linked with CSFs necessary for each goal. Options previously identified should be linked to CSFs and steps to achieve these must be identified. A matrix, map, or some other graphical representation should be developed, so that the overall strategy of the organization and the interdependencies of its various parts are easily identified.

Information System Strategic Planning

So far the organizational strategic planning process has been discussed. In the beginning of the chapter we said that if an information systems (IS) strategic plan is to be successful, it must be based on the strategic goals and CSFs of the organization. What then is the information system strategic planning (ISSP) process? How is it conducted and how is it integrated with the overall business plan of the organization?

Information System Strategic Planning Methods

There are many methods and techniques that can be used for ISSP. Martin and Leben (1989) suggest an eight-step process:

1. Performing a linkage analysis
2. Creating an overview entity-relationship enterprise model
3. Performing a technology impact analysis
4. Performing critical success factor analysis
5. Performing goal and problem analysis
6. Refining the entity-relationship diagram

7. Clustering entities into business areas
8. Establishing priorities for business area analysis

This model for ISSP stresses the importance of integrating the information systems plan with the overall business strategic plan. Primary to this model, however, is the premise that data are the focus of modern information systems technology. Thus, the information systems planning must be based on the development of an information model for the organization. Development of the information model is accomplished through entity-relationship diagrams. These diagrams portray relationships among entities in the organization. An entity is anything about which data can be stored. Examples of entities include a patient, a physician, an employee, a supplier, a physician order, and a nursing progress note. The benefit of an information model is that it clearly identifies relationships among entities and their data. This information is useful for the development of enterprise-wide data dictionaries and understanding the interfaces among entities, data, and enterprise information systems. Chapters 5 and 6 presents a thorough discussion of data administration and modeling techniques.

Another approach to ISSP is called dynamic planning by Goldberg and Sifonis (1994). In their model, Goldberg and Sifonis tightly integrate IS planning into the overall strategic business planning of the organization. In other words, information systems planning does not come after the business strategic planning process but rather is conducted within a total business strategic planning framework. Goldberg and Sifonis call this strategic alignment modeling (SAM) of the information systems structure and information systems strategy with the business structure and strategy of the organization. Within their model, alignment occurs after options have been generated in the overall strategic planning processes. The effects of each option are assessed in relation to their impact on information systems structure and information systems strategy. For example, consider the previous scenario involving Community Hospital and Health. The goal of the organization was to capture a larger share of the market. One option was to establish family practice clinics in suburban areas of the community. Obviously if this option is chosen it will have a significant impact on the information systems structure and strategy. If suburban clinics are established, communication links will be needed among all the clinics as well as the hospital. This situation will impact the design of the communication infrastructure and computer networks of the organization. It will also mean more end-users in the clinic who will need access to a help desk. Upkeep and maintenance of equipment may be affected. This option may also redefine the organizational structure within the information systems department.

Ward, Griffiths, and Whitmore (1990) suggest a strategic information systems planning process described in a framework of inputs and outputs. The inputs to the ISSP process include (1) an internal business environment assessment; (2) an external business environment assessment; (3) an internal information systems environment assessment; (4) an external information systems environment assessment. The output derived from these analyses includes (1) an information systems management strategy that manages information technology supply and demand and (2) a business information systems strategy that states how information systems will be deployed to support business functions. These authors advocate the use of various tools and techniques to arrive at the ISSP outputs. These include entity models, activity decomposition diagrams, data flow diagrams, and matrices and tables.

Another model for ISSP is presented by Boar (1993). Boar's model views the information systems organization (department) as a strategic business unit. It is looked at as a collection of related businesses having (1) a distinct mission; (2) a clear set of customers or market; (3) a set of competitors; (4) a set of products; (5) a profit and loss responsibility; and (6) a distinct management team. In his model, Boar presents a generic set of strategic planning methods and techniques and applies both the philosophy of strategic planning and its techniques to information systems planning. In other words, this model advocates using the tools and techniques employed in business planning to assess the information systems business unit, assessing the organization in which the unit resides, developing options, and developing a grand plan for the information systems unit.

All of the models have distinct benefits and drawbacks. The Martin and Leben model provides for the development of an information model that is critical to the development of enterprise-wide information systems. This model also emphasizes the importance of integrating the information systems plan with the overall business plan of the organization. However, the model does not stress evaluating the information systems unit as a critical business unit of the organization.

The strength of the Goldberg and Sifonis model is that information systems planning is intricately entwined in the total strategic business planning of the organization—that is, information systems planning does not come after the fact. It is an integral part of the process and the effects of business options are evaluated according to their impact on the information systems structure as well as strategy. This model, however, is more conceptual and does not specifically provide for information modeling techniques that are crucial to the development of enterprise-wide information systems.

The strength of the Boar model is that it emphasizes evaluation of the information systems unit from the standpoint of a critical business unit. In other words, IS is evaluated just like any other unit in the business for its strategic advantage. Other models view information systems as a support unit and do not directly assess the competitive position or value that the unit lends to the organization. Like the Goldberg and Sifonis model, however, Boar does not emphasize the importance of information modeling. The model presented by Ward, Griffiths, and Whitmore, probably more than any of the others, attempts to integrate a view of the information systems unit as a critical business unit (through internal and external information system analyses) with its function as a support unit for the enterprise. It also recognizes the importance of using tools and techniques such as CASE (computer–assisted structured engineering) and entity-relationship models for development of enterprise-wide information systems.

These models for ISSP are by no means an exhaustive list of those that exist. Certainly there are other models such as the portfolio model of Anthony (1965) and the stage model of Gibson and Nolan (1974) that was later refined by Nolan (1979). Additionally, almost every proprietary consulting firm engaged in ISSP has its own version of an ISSP model. It is probably safe to say, then, that there is no preferred ISSP model for any given organization. The chief information officer must exercise leadership in using elements from all of these models so that the best strategy for information systems planning is developed.

Developing a Customized Information Systems Planning Methodology

As was just noted, there is no dearth of planning methodologies for ISSP. Each method has its own specific philosophy, steps, techniques, and methods. Thus, the dilemma for the organization is one of choice. Does the organization choose one of the common methodologies over another, recognizing its specific limitations? Or does the organization develop a customized process and try to capture the strengths of each methodology? There is no one easy answer or choice to these questions. However, a general framework of ISSP elements is provided below. These are elements of strength that have been drawn from the various methodologies and should be considered for incorporation in any information systems strategic planning effort.

Top Management Understanding and Support

No information systems strategic planning effort will be successful without the support from executive management. Top management must not only support the ISSP process, it must also understand the implications for outcomes from such a process. Top management must understand that the ISSP process can deliver increased value to the organization from at least two perspectives. First, new business opportunities can be identified and exploited by the use of information technology that will further the competitive advantage of the organization. Second, information technologies should be developed so that the critical business functions of the organization are enhanced and maximized.

Strategic planning for information systems will result in the need for allocation of resources. It also has the potential for impacting or changing the structure or even the functions performed within an organization. Because of these far-reaching effects, it is important that the process be understood and given support from top management from the beginning. Without this support, goals and action plans developed through the planning process are not likely to be implemented. As a result, a lot of time, effort, and expense will have been invested with no tangible results.

View of Information Systems as a Strategic Business Unit

It is important that the information systems function be viewed as a critical business unit and not merely a support unit for other business units. Strategic planning techniques and analyses that are used to develop an overall business plan must also be applied to the information systems unit. For example, there should be an internal environmental assessment of the information systems unit. CSFs should be identified for the unit, a SWOT analysis should be performed in relation to the CSFs, a review of the applications portfolio should be performed, the organizational structure should be assessed, and so on. In addition, an external environmental information technology assessment should be performed. This is similar to the external environmental assessment that is performed for strategic business planning, except that the emphasis is on gaining a perspective about trends and opportunities for using information systems for competitive advantage. Like the external environmental analysis for the business, the external analysis for information systems should include looking at what competitors or others are doing. It is also advisable to look at other industries outside of health care to see how information technologies have been deployed for competitive advantage.

Integration of the Strategic Plans of the Business and Information Systems

Ideally, information systems planning should be integrated into the business strategic planning process as Goldberg and Sifonis recommend (1994). Minimally, the ISSP process should include access to information about the internal and external environments of the business. In order for any ISSP process to be successful, a thorough understanding of the organization, its business objectives, and its strategies is absolutely necessary. If the ISSP process has not been coordinated with the overall business strategic planning process, then the formal strategic plan of the organization should be made available as well as supporting documentation. Information in this documentation may need to be confirmed by additional interviews or surveys using CSF methodology or other techniques. In the worst-case scenario, there may be no business strategic plan. In this situation, the ISSP process must include mechanisms for identifying the organizational and business unit goals and CSFs. At least the information systems can support the business requirements of high-priority areas.

To develop a comprehensive and effective information systems strategic plan, there must be input about the external business environment. An understanding of the competitive forces, threats, and opportunities from a business-wide perspective will be useful in identifying areas in which information technologies can provide competitive advantage. For example, perhaps managed care is expected to be a new entrant to a specific geographical area. Perhaps, the external analysis has also shown that survival in a managed-care environment requires cost accounting as well as quality and outcome information that is integrated. Knowing that managed care is an expected critical force in the external environment would be important information for the information systems strategic planning process. In this case, the survival of the organization would be directly dependent on planning options for information systems development that would support the design of decision support systems rather than transaction systems.

Development of an Enterprisewide Information Model

The importance of the development of an enterprise-wide information model cannot be overemphasized. It is this model of entity relationships that provides the foundation for integration of all enterprise information. systems. The information model is a high-level general description of the relationship between organization entities. An entity is any person, object, or abstract concept about which data are stored. This high-level diagram and its associated data encyclopedia are further decomposed and refined into data models that support specific information systems and their associated databases. This type of modeling ensures that all enterprise-wide information systems conform to the same data definitions so that data can be easily exchanged from one information system to another within the organization.

Conclusion

There is no one sequential process for ISSP. As the discussion shows, there are several important components for a successful ISSP process. Table 4-3 provides an outline of functions that may be used for ISSP development. The functions listed in the table should not necessarily be performed sequentially. For example, the internal and external information systems analysis can be performed concurrently with the development of the enterprise-wide information model. Other activities may also be performed concurrently, such as the identification of organization strategic goals and thrusts. The formulation of the process of ISSP is very organization specific and depends on the culture of the organization, the timetable for strategic planning, and the amount of resources, both human and financial, that can be devoted to the project.

Once the information systems strategic planning process has concluded, a formal document must be developed. This document is essential in providing guidance to information systems development activities. The document plan should clearly set forth the information needs of the organization and demonstrate how information system objectives support the strategic thrusts of the organization. Table 4-4 is an outline for an information systems plan. Again, this is a generic outline. Actual information systems plan content and format will vary from organization to organization.

Table 4-3.   Elements of Development of an Information Systems Strategic Plan

Identify key organizational strategic goals and/or critical success factors.

Link organizational goals to information system requirements.

Identify information needs of the organization through the development of an information model.

Prioritize information system requirements.

Perform an internal information system analysis.

Perform an external information system analysis.

Evaluate the gap between information system requirements and current information systems environment.

Identify long-term information system objectives.

Identify long-term information system strategies to obtain objectives.

Identify resource requirements to implement strategies (i.e., people, technologies, costs, and time frame).

Forecast expenditures required to obtain strategic objectives.

Table 4-4.   Generic Outline of an Information Systems Strategic Plan

Executive Summary:	Provides a quick overview of the progress that has been made; the critical issues that the organization is facing, the information system objectives and strategies, and a summary of the key factors and support needed for success. A summary of the cost of plan implementation is also provided.
Planning Process:	Provides a description of the planning process and how the critical success factors or strategic thrusts of the organization are considered by the plan.
Function Statement:	Provides the mission and vision statements for the information systems department.
Environmental Assessment:	Provides an overview of the current status of information systems. Includes internal and external issues that will impact information systems. Assesses the organizational critical success factors or strategic objectives vis-à-vis the current information system environment. The analysis should provide the information necessary to establish the direction and priorities of the information systems plan. May also include organization information model in an appendix.

Table 4-4.   *(cont.)*

Long-term Objectives:	Includes organization, application, hardware, and network strategies that are necessary to meet the organization's information requirements. Prioritization of information system projects.
Financial Projections:	At least a 3-year forecast of required expenditures.
Appendices:	Information model(s); results of data gathering; detailed information architecture graphics, sample survey instruments, etc.

The Health Information Manager's Role in Strategic IS Planning

It is highly likely that the health information manager will be asked to participate in both the overall business planning strategy and the information systems strategic planning process. Activities associated with the external analysis of the environment and external analysis of information technologies require exhaustive data retrieval efforts. The health information manager possesses a skill in data retrieval and knowledge of databases that can be helpful to these external analyses efforts. Therefore, it is probable that the health information manager will be called on to be a member of one of the task forces associated with the external analyses.

In addition to the external analyses, the health information manager can provide essential skills and knowledge to the internal business analysis effort. The health information manager has access to a number of data sources that would be useful to the data-gathering aspects of this activity. In addition, the health information manager could function effectively in the development of interview protocols and surveys to assess the internal nature of the business. Knowledge of the clinical aspects of health-care delivery in the organization and related information needs would make the health information manager a valuable member of the interview team. Thus, the health information manager should be prepared to function as a task force member on an internal analysis effort.

In addition to the business strategic planning effort, the health information manager should be included in various aspects of the internal and external analysis of the information systems unit. Again, skills in data access and knowledge of information sources will make the health information manager a valuable team member in assessing trends and opportunities for the deployment of information technologies. Certainly the health information manager should also be included in activities relating to the development of the enterprise-wide information model. Knowledge about the clinical aspects of health-care delivery, entities, and their relationships will prove useful in the development of any information model.

Thus, it is evident that the health information manager has a significant role to play in both the business and information systems strategic planning processes. As noted previously, the strategic planning process is a critical function within the professional practice domain of information engineering.

Summary

- The design of enterprise information systems should be tied to the strategic planning efforts of the organization.
- The strategic planning effort for information systems must be supported by top management of the organization in order to be successful.
- Both internal and external analyses are necessary to develop an information systems strategic plan that supports the strategic thrusts of the organization.
- When preparing an information systems plan to support organization-wide functions, it is also necessary to view the information systems department as a strategic business unit.

Review Questions

1. Why is top management support critical for the success of an information systems strategic planning effort?
2. Why are both internal and external analyses necessary for development of a strategic information systems plan? What might the consequences be if one of these analyses were not done?

3. What is the difference between an operational plan and a strategic plan for information services? Why is this difference important?

4. How would you go about integrating the information systems plan with the enterprise strategic plan?

5. Provide some examples of how information systems might improve the competitive position of an organization.

Enrichment Activities

1. Review an information systems strategic plan from a local health-care facility. Are the components of the plan consistent with those mentioned in this chapter? If not, what components are missing or added? Evaluate whether or not the information systems plan adequately supports the strategic objectives of the organization.

2. Interview a chief information officer at a local health-care facility regarding information systems strategic planning. What methodology did the enterprise use to develop the information systems plan? Is this methodology consistent with the material discussed in this chapter? What barriers did the organization have to overcome to develop an information systems plan? Would the CIO proceed the same way in a similar situation? What would the CIO do differently to make the process stronger?

References

Anthony, R. N. (1965). *Planning and control: A framework for analysis*. Cambridge, MA: Harvard University Press.

Boar, B. H. (1993). *The art of strategic planning for information technology*. New York: John Wiley & Sons.

Gibson, C. F., and Nolan, R. L. (1974, January–February). Managing the four stages of EDP growth. *Harvard Business Review*.

Goldberg, B., and Sifonis, J. G. (1994). *Dynamic planning: The art of managing beyond tomorrow*. New York: Oxford University Press.

Martin, J., and Leben, J. (1989). *Strategic information planning methodologies*, 2nd ed. Englewood Cliffs, NJ: Prentice Hall.

Nolan, R. L. (1979, March–April). Managing the crisis in data processing. *Harvard Business Review.*

Porter, M. (1980). *Competitive strategy: Techniques for analyzing industries and competitors.* New York: Free Press.

Porter, M. (1985). *Competitive strategy: Techniques for analyzing industries and competitors.* New York: Free Press.

Rockart, John (1979, March–April). Chief executives define their own data needs. *Harvard Business Review*, p. 80.

Ward, J., Griffiths, P., and Whitmore, K. P. (1990). *Strategic planning for information systems.* Chichester, England: John Wiley & Sons.

Chapter 5

Design and Development of Information Systems

Learning Objectives

After completing of this chapter, the learner should be able to:

1. Discuss the stages in the traditional systems development life cycle.
2. Evaluate the strengths and weaknesses of the traditional systems development life cycle.
3. Describe methodologies that can be used to quickly design and develop information systems.
4. State the purpose of data modeling.
5. Discuss the benefits of using the data modeling process in the design of information systems.
6. Define the customary steps in the data modeling process.
7. Describe the differences between conceptual, external, and internal data models.
8. Differentiate between entities, attributes, and relationships in a data model.
9. List and describe the contents of a conceptual data model.
10. Describe the purpose and various functions of CASE tools.
11. Distinguish the various notations in a data model diagram.

Key Terms

Attribute

CASE Tools

Conceptual Data Model

Data Modeling

Entity

Entity-Relationship Diagram

External Data Model

Internal Data Model

Joint Application Design

Rapid Application Development Tools

Systems Development Life Cycle

Introduction

As discussed in Chapter 4, the strategic planning process is a critical first step in the development of an information systems strategy for an enterprise. However, you are probably asking, "What happens after the strategic planning process is completed? How are the required information systems developed to support the information needs of the enterprise?" This chapter provides answers to these questions. The chapter first presents an overview of the traditional methodology used in systems design and development called the systems development life cycle (SDLC). This method has been useful over many years, but the pressures for quicker and more integrated development of information systems has prompted the growth of new methodologies. Therefore, this chapter focuses on the use of newer methodologies for design and development of information systems.

Traditional Systems Development Life Cycle

The traditional method for information system development has followed a set of specified stages called the **systems development life cycle** (SDLC). The SDLC has been a particularly appropriate methodology when information systems have been developed in house by the health-care organization. The stages of the life cycle vary somewhat depending on the methodology used. However, all methodologies contain stages relating to the initiation, development, implementation, and operation of the system. For our purposes, we define the traditional SDLC as consisting of four stages: (1) system initiation, (2) system development, (3) system implementation, and (4) system operation. The learner can readily see that just like any other life cycle, information systems development has a beginning point (initiation), a growth stage (development), a birth stage (implementation), and a maturation stage (operation). Each of these stages may have several phases or steps. Table 5-1 presents an outline of the normal steps within each stage of the developmental life cycle.

While the life cycle approach is very systematic, it has several drawbacks. First, the approach is not wholistic—that is, it does not include the development of information systems based on an enterprise information model. Although the actual steps of the development process make sense and can produce an excellent operational product, the SDLC does not ensure the appropriate integration of information systems from an enterprise perspective. As we know, the lack of an integrated approach to information systems development critically undermines the development of useful information systems in today's competitive environment. Begin-

Table 5-1. System Development Life Cycle Stages

Initiation	• Request for system development
	• Requirements and systems analysis
Development	• System design
	• Specification of functions
	• Coding of computer program(s)
	• Testing of system
Implementation	• Development of system documentation
	• User training
	• System conversion
Operation	• Operation of the system
	• System maintenance
	• System changes/upgrades

ning information systems development by using newer methods, such as data modeling, helps to alleviate this problem.

A second weakness of the SDLC is that the approach is extremely time-consuming. The time it takes to go through the stages of project initiation to project implementation can take many months, if not years! It is not uncommon to find systems development backlogs in health-care enterprises of 2 to 3 years. Other methodologies such as prototyping and rapid application development (RAD) tools help reduce this drawback.

Another drawback of the SDLC is that there frequently is not sufficient emphasis on end-user input in the development process. Analysts will usually meet and talk with end-users about their application needs. The analysts translate these needs into various diagrams. These diagrams are helpful communication devices for programmers, but end-users frequently cannot understand them. The result is often that misinterpretations between the analysts and end-users are not discovered until well into system development or system implementation. Newer techniques, such as the use of rapid prototyping, scenario-based development, and joint application development (JAD), help to minimize this drawback.

Another deficiency of the SDLC approach is that frequently application development is performed in a vacuum with little or no consideration of the overlap between other existing applications and current projects. The result is often poor integration among systems and unnecessary duplication. As we know, the health-care industry has witnessed dramatic changes in the information required by customers in a managed-care environment. Although health-care enterprises may have data that will satisfy these information requirements, these data are usually "locked" into separate applications and are not easily retrievable in an integrated fashion. Thus, systems developed using a traditional life cycle have tended to be inflexible.

In the past few years, methods and tools have been developed to overcome many of the difficulties associated with the traditional SDLC. Foremost has been the development of the concept of information engineering. While there are several methodologies used to implement this concept, the principle of information engineering is based on a holistic view of an enterprise's information requirements. This includes how the information is managed and controlled. Thus, the emphasis is to develop systems that support organizational processes and information needs of the organization. Such basic processes and information requirements are not likely to change dramatically. For example, a health maintenance organization requires clinical data, inventory data, accounting data, marketing data, human resources data, and so on. A change in organizational structure of the enterprise will not change the need for these data. Thus, if information systems are designed around the enterprise information needs and generic processes, the systems will be flexible and able to accommodate changes in organizational structure and/or changes in emphasis of the external environment.

New Approaches and New Tools

Over the past several years, new approaches and tools have been developed to overcome the difficulties encountered with the traditional SDLC. Some of these are described below and fall into the general area of information engineering approaches and techniques.

Development of the Enterprise Information Model

Probably the most significant approach away from the traditional SDLC is the trend to begin information systems design with the development of an enterprise information model. Unlike a specific applications development project, which is extremely detailed, the enterprise information model focuses on the "big picture" of the organization's information needs. The modeling process considers the goals of the enterprise, identifies data requirements, identifies activities or processes to be supported, and sets priorities for implementation. The enterprise information model categorizes data into groups and identifies the relationships between these groups. Information models are generally represented in a schematic called an **entity-relationship diagram** (ERD). The following scenario provides a simple example of how an enterprise information model may be developed:

A
n outpatient clinic treats several patients per day. Each patient is seen by a primary-care provider. Each patient may also have ancillary services performed including laboratory, radiology, or other types of tests.

If we were to develop an information model for the outpatient clinic based on this scenario, we would first identify the various processes and groups of data required to support each process. The processes in this example would include patient registration; patient examination by a clinician such as a physician, nurse practitioner, or physician assistant; and the performance of diagnostic tests. In this case, we would need a group of data about the patient to support the registration, examination, and diagnostic processes. This may consist of the patient's name, birthdate, medical record number, and sex. We would also need a group of data about the visit. This may consist of the date of the visit, the time of the visit, the chief complaint, the final diagnosis, and the disposition of the patient. We would also need a group of data about the primary-care provider who saw the patient. In this case, the data may consist of the clinician name and clinician identification number. Finally, we would need a group of data about the tests that the patient received. These data may include the name of the test and the identification number of the test. Thus, using this simple example we have begun to build an information model for the outpatient clinic. Later in this chapter we will learn how such an information model is diagrammed using special application software called computer-aided software engineering (CASE) tools.

Notice that this information model is application independent, which means the data do not depend on a specific application such as a billing application, accounting application, or medical records application. Rather the data that make up each of these groups can be used by all applications. This concept is called data independence and is important in the design of enterprise databases to ensure minimal redundancy of data and standardized definitions for each data element.

Naturally an enterprise information model will be much more complex than the one just described. In a real enterprise there are perhaps hundreds of data groupings. Once an enterprise information model is developed for the enterprise, all individual applications development is then based on the enterprise information model.

Computer-Aided Software Engineering Tools

Development of information systems from an integrated perspective relies heavily on charts and graphics such as data flow and entity-relationship diagrams, data dictionaries, and other types of tables and schematics. These types of graphics are necessary in order to track interrelationships among data and organizational processes. An example of a fairly simple entity-relationship diagram (ERD) appears in Figure 5-1.

An organization may have hundreds and perhaps thousands of entity-relationship diagrams alone! As would be expected, such graphics are next to impossible to manually draw and to update. Therefore, a number of software tools have been developed that help with system analysis and design and the creation of such diagrams and models. These tools are referred to as computer-aided software engineering (CASE) tools.

There are several categories of **CASE tools.** Some of these tools are designed to help with the initial analysis and requirements definition of a system, for example, data flow diagrams (DFD) and structure charts. Such diagrams and charts identify the processes of an organization and document the flow of data from one process to another. This is an important step in the development of the data model. You must first understand the processes that an organization performs before you can identify the information requirements for those processes. The DFD in Figure 5-7 (later in this chapter) documents four processes that occur during a patient clinic visit: registering a patient, gathering initial clinical data about the patient visit, treating the patient, and performing tests on the patient. These processes are identified in the DFD by rounded rectangles. Near each process is the method used to carry it out. For example, in order to register a patient, a registration screen is used. To compile initial information about the patient, an admit screen is used. Note that the entity "patient" is notated using a rectangle, and the database, "patient file," where all data are ultimately stored, is notated using an open rectangle.

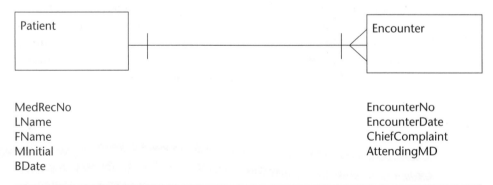

Figure 5-1. Simple Entity-Relationship (ER) Diagram

There are also CASE tools that assist the design team in prototyping a system. Prototyping a system allows for maximal user input and helps to speed up the development process. Prototyping is an iterative process where the analyst and end-users work together to develop the external features of a system. Such features may include the design of screens, interaction between screens, and reports. A working prototype is a front-end model that simulates how system features will function once the actual product is developed. A prototype does not usually include a working database or actual program application code, but merely provides the "touch and feel" of the system to be designed.

To speed up the development process, there are also tools to make programming and testing of programming code faster. Such CASE tools are normally referred to as coding tools and include fourth-generation languages (4GL), screen generators, code generators, and program templates.

Rapid Application Development Tools

In addition to the CASE tools that assist with the modeling of data and actual programming and testing of code, **rapid application development (RAD) tools** help with the prototyping of a system. As mentioned earlier, prototyping is an iterative process whereby the end-user and analyst work together to develop a model of the proposed system. An iterative process is one in which the user and analyst work together developing parts of the prototype one at a time. Each time one part of the system is developed, the user and analyst review it and test it to determine if the functions and features of the system are correct. For example, in developing a prototype of a medication order-entry system, the user and analyst might first design the initial input screen for the system. The screen would be developed using a prototyping tool such as Microsoft Visual Basic. Once the initial screen is designed, its features and functions would be evaluated by the end-user and analyst. Any problems could be corrected immediately before proceeding to design subsequent input and output screens. This iterative process would continue until a mockup of the finished product was developed.

Such an iterative process has several benefits. First, it increases end-user involvement in the analysis and development process. Second, a working prototype of the system can be developed quickly, usually in a matter of days instead of months! Third, the prototype provides the look and feel of the real system to eventually be developed. This allows the user a better opportunity to assess whether or not the system as designed will provide essential support to the work task involved.

Joint Application Design

Joint application design (JAD) is a technique that is used in place of the traditional systems and analysis methods of interviewing and surveying end-users and observing work tasks. JAD provides an opportunity for substantial end-user input as well as speeding the development process. With the JAD method, a group of end-users, analysts, and technical experts meet over a period of several days to analyze information requirements and identify information system alternatives. The premise underlying JAD methodology is that a group of individuals working together at the same time can perform analysis and identify system features faster and better than individuals working independently through the traditional sequential analysis process. Many times prototyping tools are also used in conjunction with the JAD process. This combination of tools and methods provides for a very fast analysis and design process.

Use of New Approaches for Analysis and Design

The previous section of this chapter discusses both the traditional method of information system development (the SDLC) and newer approaches that are being used to speed up and integrate information systems development. The professional model of practice presented in Figure 1-3 in Chapter 1 suggests that an important role of the health information manager is to participate in data modeling tasks. Therefore, the emphasis for the rest of this chapter is on data modeling concepts and techniques, tools, and methods.

Data Modeling

As we have learned, an important part of the information engineering domain is **data modeling**. Once the strategic planning efforts for the organization are completed, the information systems required to support the strategic thrusts of the enterprise can be determined. A good example is the following scenario that describes the outcomes of the strategic planning for a 350-bed acute-care facility:

Mt. Pleasant Hospital has just completed a strategic planning process. One outcome of the planning was the generation of critical success factors for the hospital. These included:

1. Provide quality care.
2. Have efficient operations.
3. Develop good physician relations.
4. Obtain optimal reimbursement and case mix.
5. Have a high perception of efficiency and service by various constituents.

These critical success factors were identified as the limited number of areas in which results, if they are satisfactory, will ensure successful competitive performance for the hospital. Subsequent to the planning process, the hospital's information systems committee began the process of integrating the long-range information systems plan with the business plan of the institution. An integral part of this planning effort was to develop information systems that supported the monitoring and achievement of the critical success factors of the institution. To determine the types of information systems that were needed to support these critical success factors, the committee developed an information systems planning matrix. A sample of this matrix for the quality-of-care critical success factors is provided in Table 5-2.

As Table 5-2 displays, several measures for monitoring quality of care were identified, including the percentage of patient complications, mortality/morbidity rates, adverse patient-care events, medication errors, patient complaints. For each measure, an information system and its function was identified that would provide the needed data and support to help achieve the quality-of-care critical success factor. This type of matrix was expanded and used to identify the general class of information systems needed to support all of the other critical success factors.

As the above scenario clearly describes, Mt. Pleasant Hospital needs a variety of information systems to support what it has identified as its critical success factors to stay competitive in the marketplace. After identifying the general classes of information systems needed, one of the first steps in planning for these systems is the process of data modeling.

Table 5-2. Quality-of-Care CSF and Information System Matrix

CSF	Measures	Information System	Functional Requirements
1. Quality of Care	% Complications	Diagnostic index	Tracking Trends Calculations Analysis
		Incident reports	
	Mortality & Morbidity Rates	Diagnostic index	Tracking Trends Calculations Analysis Projections
		Infection control	
		Incident reports	
	Adverse patient events	Diagnostic index	Tracking Trends Calculations Analysis Projections
		Incident reports	
	Patient complaints	Satisfaction survey	Tracking Trends Calculations Analysis Projections
		Incident reports	

A Definition of Data Modeling

A model is usually defined as a small copy or imitation of an existing object. A model is usually a representation of something that is to be copied. For example, an architect who is designing a new wing of a clinic or hospital will develop a model of the building. The model, which is a small scale of the proposed building, is used to show clients what the product will look like when it is finished. Other common models that are representations of existing objects include model airplanes, model trains, and model ships.

Data modeling and the development of enterprise databases must be based on a strategic plan for development of organizational information systems. Before any information systems developmental effort is started, it is essential to understand what data the business needs. Therefore, it is necessary to study what these business data are and how they relate to each other. The data modeling process actually is a methodology that aids in this identification. The data model is based on the business strategic plan and provides a graphical picture of the business data needs. It is helpful in developing the general information systems master plan for the organization. This master information systems plan lays out all the application and database requirements and sets out the priorities for each of these. Applications and databases are then developed on a priority basis. In order for databases and applications to be developed, however, there must be a significant level of detail describing the data and the purposes of the applications. The data modeling process assists in the development of this detail.

Like the architect's model that is used as a prototype for the actual structure to be built, the data model is used as the plan for building complex organizational databases. All too often, however, the development of databases and associated applications is not planned in sufficient detail to ensure successful outcomes. In order for good applications and databases to be developed, information systems professionals must take the time to develop useful models. These models should describe how data flow, the requirements and usage of the data, and the attributes of the data. Therefore, data modeling is a first essential step in ensuring successful database and application development. Figure 5-2 represents data requirements of an emergency department encounter.

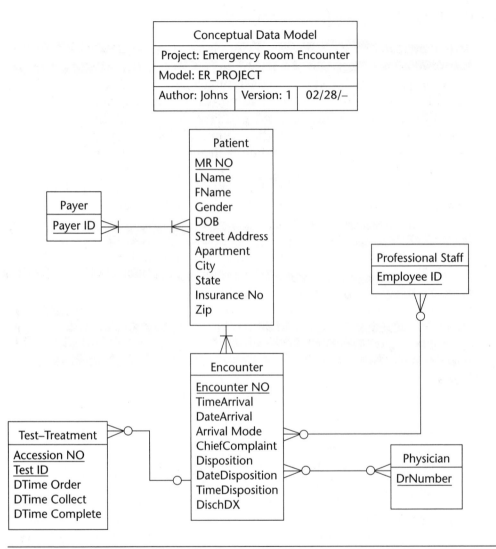

Figure 5-2.   Conceptual Data Model of Emergency Department

Categories of Data Models

There are three types of data models: conceptual, external, and internal data models. The **conceptual data model,** sometimes called the conceptual schema, defines the database requirements of the enterprise in a single database description. There is only one conceptual data model maintained for the enterprise that represents the information needs of the organization. The development of the conceptual data model is an integral part of a top-down planning process.

The conceptual data model is used as the basis for the development of both the external and internal data models. The **external data model,** sometimes called the logical data model, is the view of the data by a specific group of users or by a specific processing application. As an example, Mt. Pleasant Hospital would have one conceptual data model. However, groups of users, such as the admitting personnel, nursing service, health information management department, human resources, and central supply, would each have their own view of the data model. Each of these views would represent the specific data flows and requirements for each group. It is important to remember, though, that all external data models are derived from the enterprise-wide conceptual model. Figure 5-3 depicts the relationship between the conceptual data model and the users' views or external data models.

As Figure 5-3 shows, each external data model is an overlapping subset of the enterprise-wide data model. The conceptual data model is initially general in nature. As more and more user views or external models are developed from a bottom-up process, the conceptual data model becomes increasingly refined and detailed.

The **internal data model,** sometimes called the physical data model, depicts how the data are physically represented in the database. The development of the internal data model is concerned with data structures, file organizations, and mechanisms and techniques to most efficiently store data and make use of the database system. The development of the internal data model is the responsibility of information systems personnel with no interaction with users. This is unlike the development of the conceptual and external data models, which require input from end-users. The emphasis of this chapter is on understanding principles associated with conceptual and external data models since the health information manager is likely to be involved in developing them.

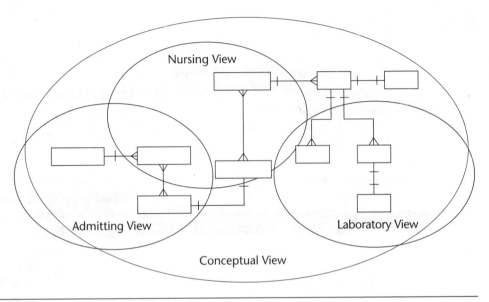

Figure 5-3.   Relationship between Conceptual and External Views

Content of a Conceptual or Business Data Model

Now that the importance of developing an enterprise or business data model has been established, you might be asking, "What constitutes a business or conceptual data model? What documentation is contained in this model?" The contents will depend on the modeling style and tools used to develop the model and will also depend on the needs of the organization. However, it is probably safe to say that a business data model usually contains the following elements (Brown, 1993):

- Diagrams
- Glossary
- Narratives
- Access patterns

As mentioned previously, a data model is a representation of the data that an enterprise needs to support its essential functions. The model depicts these data and their relationships among each other through a series of diagrams. The diagrams, in essence, provide a picture of the data needs of the enterprise. The notations or symbols used in the diagrams will vary depending on the modeling methodology or style that is used. For example, some modeling styles use entity-relationship diagrams (ERD) whereas others may use bubble charts and information engineering (IE) diagrams. Regardless of the method used, the diagrams will usually show the names of entities (or things) about which data are stored and the relationship among these entities. An explanation of entities is presented in the next section of this chapter.

A second element of the data model is the glossary. Depending on the methodology used, this is sometimes referred to as the catalog or data dictionary. Every name that is documented on the data model diagram should be defined in a glossary. For example, if the diagram shows the name "physician order," the glossary should provide a definition of what constitutes a physician order. If the diagram shows the name "patient," the glossary should provide a definition of patient. The data elements that compose or make up the entity of "patient" might appear like that in Figure 5-4. In this figure, the data elements of "Lname," "Fname," Minitial," "Sex," and "Bdate" constitute the entity "patient."

In addition to diagrams and a glossary, the data model includes narratives to help explain what the diagram and glossary mean. Narratives are useful adjuncts to communicate to both users and developers what the data model diagram is trying to convey.

Name: Patient

Code: Pt

Description: This entity describes the demographics of a patient treated by the Emergency Department

Attribute Name	Code	Type	Length
Last Name	Lname	Character	20
First Name	Fname	Character	20
Middle Initial	Minitial	Character	1
Birth Date	Bdate	Date	6

Figure 5-4. Glossary Description

Statements about access patterns are sometimes included in the data model documentation. It is important for the physical database developers to know what data are accessed, how often these data are accessed, and in what order they are accessed. Knowing this information is critical for planning for optimal response and transaction times.

The above documentation elements taken together constitute the enterprise data model. This documentation is essential to developing an enterprise-wide view of the organization's information needs. In addition, the documentation provides a communication mechanism among designers, users, and developers that promotes basic understanding of the business information processes and uses. The compilation of the data model documentation also provides the basis for optimal enterprise-wide database design.

Data Modeling Methods and Styles

There is not one, single, standard data modeling style or method. The method chosen by an enterprise will be based on its needs, the training and knowledge of its information systems designers, and the culture of the organization. Thus, the notation and language used (particularly in diagrams) may vary greatly from one data modeling method to another. Popular data modeling methods include the Chen entity-relationship (ER) style, the information engineering (IE) method, and Nijssen's information analysis methodology (NIAM). The Chen ER method was first published in 1976. Since that time there have been many extensions to the notations and meanings used in this style. Information engineering was developed by Clive Finkelstein and first published in 1981. Many vendors of CASE tools support the IE methodology. NIAM was first introduced during the early 1970s. Since then, NIAM has continually evolved and is one of the more popular methods used in Europe. Figure 5-5 provides a comparison between these various notational styles.

For some development teams, the structured approach to systems analysis using diagrams and tools such as the data flow diagram (DFD), hierarchy charts, and structured data diagrams is considered to be part of the data modeling process. Regardless of the methodology, there are several common concepts shared among all of the popular styles. First, each of these methods is based on the premise that all information is based on entities or things and that there are relationships among these entities.

CHEN-ER Diagram

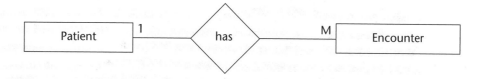

Information Engineering Diagram

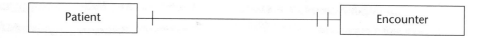

Bubble Diagram

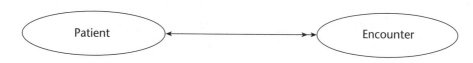

Figure 5-5. Comparison of Conceptual Data Model Notations

This basic premise is operationalized through the use of three principal structural elements found in the data model diagram: entities, relationships, and attributes.

An **entity** is a person, place, thing, or concept about which data are gathered. For example, a patient is a person about which facts are recorded. A visit to the emergency department of a hospital is a concept about which facts are recorded. An operating room is a place about which data are recorded. For any given enterprise there likely will be hundreds and probably thousands of entities about which data are recorded.

An **attribute** is a fact or piece of information describing an entity. Consider the visit of a patient to the emergency department, for example. Certain data (attributes) are collected about the patient when the patient comes to the emergency department and certain data (attributes) are collected about each emergency room encounter. For instance, a patient's gender or sex is an attribute of the entity "patient." A medical record number is also an attribute of the entity "patient" because it provides a fact about a patient. The chief complaint of a patient arriving in the emergency department would be an attribute of an emergency department encounter because it provides a fact about an emergency department visit. The date of arrival to the emergency department would be another example of an attribute of a emergency department encounter.

In addition to entities and attributes, every data modeling method shows relationships among entities. For example, the entity "patient" is related to "emergency department encounter" because every person coming to the emergency department has an emergency department encounter.

The data model diagram names each entity, defines each entity by its attributes, and shows relationships among various entities. For example, Figure 5-6 is a simple ER diagram showing the relationship between the entity "patient" and the entity "emergency department encounter." In this notation, entities are drawn as rectangles and the relation is drawn as a line connecting the entities. The attributes for each entity are listed near the entity to which they correspond. In this example, the entity "patient"

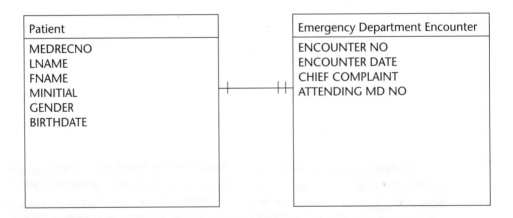

Figure 5-6. Relationship between Patient and Emergency Department Encounter

has the attributes of MedRecNo, LName, FName, MInitial, Gender, and Birthdate. The entity "emergency department encounter" has the attributes of Encounter No, Encounter Date, Chief Complaint, and Attending MD No.

Steps in the Data Modeling Process

Now that the concepts of data modeling and various styles have been introduced, a logical question is, "How is the data model developed?" Several steps are essential to ensure the success of the data modeling process: (1) formation of the data modeling/planning team; (2) determination of the planning tools that will be used; (3) studying user requirements and defining these through the use of data modeling diagrams; and (4) development of the database design.

Formation of the Data Modeling Team

The data modeling process is a significant work effort. Depending on the project, a data modeling project can take from weeks to months to complete. Therefore, for any data modeling effort, a data modeling team must be organized. Ideally the team will be composed of user representatives, information systems analysts, and database specialists. Because of the significant time and labor effort, the data modeling project, particularly if it is an enterprise-wide thrust, must have the support of top management. The data modeling effort crosses departmental boundaries, affecting several organizational divisions. Therefore, there must be a clear understanding about the purpose, expected outcomes, and benefits of the project. These must be communicated to all the sections of the enterprise that will be affected so that their cooperation and participation in the process can be ensured.

Selection of Data Modeling Tools

The identification of data and the design of the relationship among data is a monumental effort. The number of entities to be identified, their various attributes, and their relationship to each other is a huge "bookkeeping" task. Fortunately, as we have already seen, there are CASE and other automated tools that help with documenting information about data and assist with the graphical design of data relationships.

As we have already learned, CASE software is an application that helps create and compile various types of analysis tools. For example, CASE software will help developers create data flow diagrams (DFD), data dictionaries (DD), entity-relationship diagrams (ERD), and other charts, tables, and schematics. Developers interact with CASE software using a graphic user interface (GUI) to create diagrams like we saw in Figure 5-6 that represent data of an enterprise and explain interrelationships among these data. Figure 5-7 depicts another type of graphical picture developed by CASE software. It is called a data flow diagram or DFD.

In this DFD, databases where data are stored are represented by an open rectangle; data flows or movement of data from one process or point to another are represented by arrows; transformations of, or operations on, data are represented by rounded rectangles; and external entities are represented by rectangles.

An important aspect of CASE software is that it creates an electronic depository where all diagrams, charts, tables, and data dictionaries are stored. This feature allows developers easy access to data model diagrams

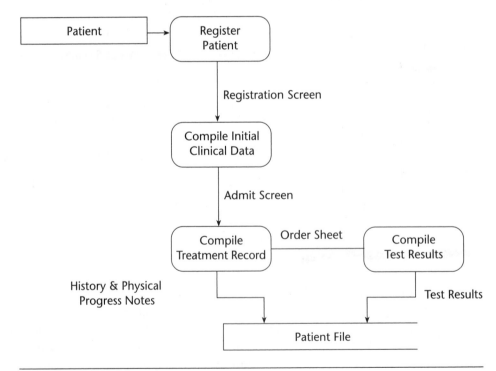

Figure 5-7. Sample Data Flow Diagram

and documentation and permits easy information retrieval or update of these diagrams when needed.

Selection of CASE software tools is based on the needs of the design team and the function preferred or required by the project. Even though such CASE tools usually cost several thousand dollars, their cost is outweighed by the multiple benefits they provide. CASE software improves the efficiency, accuracy, and completeness of the data model (and system analysis) process. One study indicated that productivity development increased by 15 percent when CASE software was used in system development effort (Perry, 1993). In today's environment, without such a computerized software application, it would be impossible to manually create, catalog, and store the hundreds and sometimes thousands of charts and diagrams associated with the development of an enterprise-wide data model.

In addition to its obvious advantage of convenience for developers in creating diagrams and charts, CASE applications provide an effective mechanism to update data model diagrams, charts, and tables. Because all diagrams, charts, tables, and dictionaries are stored electronically in a central repository, it is easy for developers to access information about them or update documentation as needed. Another important benefit of CASE application software is that it imposes standardization. When used on an enterprise-wide basis, all development efforts use the same type of notation and documentation style. Additionally, since all development projects draw on and contribute to the same central repository of information, the CASE software allows for automatic consistency checks. Thus, there is no duplication and errors are reduced significantly.

Defining User Requirements

One of the most important steps in the data modeling process is the identification of user requirements. The data modeling team works with end-users to (1) identify the scope of the project (i.e., database and applications), (2) collect data about the processes to be automated, and (3) document data requirements.

Identifying the Scope of the Project   Identifying the scope of the project is critical to success. Frequently, end-users will have unrealistic expectations of the outcomes of the project. Therefore, it is the responsibility of the development team to work with the users to define reasonable expectations and boundaries for the project. This is usually accomplished through a series of initial meetings with representative end-users and the development team.

During these meetings, end-users are queried in general about their expectations for the proposed system. Usually, end-users will identify outcomes that encompass more than the development of one system. It is imperative that all subsystems and interrelated systems be identified and then priorities assigned for development. For example, a group of end-users from the health information management department of a clinic met with the development team to discuss the design of a chart-tracking system. Once the meeting got underway, it was obvious that the end-users expected more than a chart-tracking system. What they were describing was a system that kept track of not only the location of patient medical records but also the number of documentation deficiencies for each chart by each physician and a running log of correspondence requests. In this case, it was necessary for the development team to help the end-users identify the differences among each of these systems, how these systems might overlap, and priorities for development.

Collecting Data about the User Requirements Once the scope of the project has been identified, the development team concentrates on collecting data about the processes for which a new system will be developed. Data collection tools will vary depending on the type and scope of the project. Traditional data-gathering techniques such as one-on-one interviews, focus groups, questionnaires, and observation are used. However, as we have already learned, these traditional approaches have significant drawbacks. Therefore, consideration should be given to the JAD and RAD techniques previously discussed.

Identifying the user requirements and arriving at a common understanding of the processes to be automated is a difficult task. More often than not, programs that are developed that do not satisfy user needs are the result of users poorly articulating their needs and/or analysts misconstruing what these needs are. Therefore, it is imperative that the development team use an iterative process to clarify with the users what outcomes are really expected. This iterative process can be accomplished through JAD and RAD techniques. Needs are also identified by documenting the processes to be automated through some type of notation and iteratively reviewing the notation with the user. Frequently this notation is the data flow diagram (DFD) as we saw in Figure 5-7.

How do we begin to clearly articulate end-user needs and the specifications of the system? One popular tool for collecting data from users is the face-to-face interview. In the face-to-face interview the development team interviews individual users or a group of users about the problems to be solved by the new system. The interview technique has several advantages. First, it provides end-users with an opportunity to describe their needs. This participation helps to encourage cooperation and develop a sense of ownership for the project by the end-users. Second, the interview process provides the development team with the opportunity to probe users about what it is that they believe they need and what problems the new system is expected to solve.

The design team may use either unstructured, semistructured, structured, or scenario-based interview techniques. In an unstructured technique, neither the questions nor their responses are specified in advance. An unstructured interview may begin by simply asking users to "Describe what you think the functions of the new system should be." Although this approach can allow for detailed probing of the user about requirements, it also has the drawback of potentially leading the interview on unnecessary tangents. In fact, the process may be so unstructured that the real issues involving system specifications are never fully addressed.

The totally structured interview is one in which the questions and the responses are fixed ahead of time. An example of a structured interview question would be asking the end-users, "Do you use a microcomputer to do your job tasks?" This question has a structured response; either the end-user responds "yes" or the end-user responds "no." While structured questions are helpful in gathering data about facts, they are less useful in probing about functional specifications. Certainly the structured interview technique is not a useful tool to determine the data flow of an organization where iterative and validation techniques should be used.

The semistructured interview combines the strengths and minimizes the weaknesses of the totally unstructured and structured interview techniques. In a semistructured interview questions are prepared in advance. It is important that these questions be asked in a sensible order so that information about user requirements is gathered that minimizes incorrect assumptions. For the most part, these questions should be context-free and open-ended. One way the semistructured interview may begin is by saying, "List the things that you want the new information system to provide or do and list the things that you don't want the information system to provide or do." For example, in the quality-of-care example from Mt. Pleasant Hospital, end-users might say they want the information system to provide tracking of adverse patient events, provide projections and trends, interface with external databases to provide comparative trends, perform statistical analyses, provide real-time data, and have a graphical user interface (GUI). In this same example, end-users may say that they don't want the information system to be microcomputer based, they don't want it to be menu driven, and they don't want data from it to be shared by other systems. Once the end-users have developed these lists, the developmental team can ask more probing questions. For example, the team may ask the end-users, "What do you mean by adverse patient events?" or "What do you mean by tracking an adverse patient event?" It is important that the development team clarify and reclarify with end-users what they mean in order to avoid ambiguity. Through many question iterations, the development team and the end-users will begin to develop a picture of the system specifications.

Gause and Weinberg (1989) provide a good list of context-free questions. Context-free questions are questions that, because of their general nature, can be asked in any developmental effort. Some of the questions that can be asked of the end-user include:

- Who is the true client that this product is going to serve?
- What is a highly successful solution really worth to this client?
- What is the real reason for solving this problem?
- How much time can this project afford to take?
- What is the trade-off between time, value, and cost?
- Is there already an information solution that exists for this problem?
- What problems does this system solve?
- What problems might this system create?
- What is the environment in which this information system must operate?
- Are you the right person to answer these questions?
- Who else should I interview?

The scenario-based interview method has become a popular technique in the last few years to help in determining system requirements. Using this method, the end-user is either presented with a case that represents a current situation or is asked to develop the scenario. The end-user then responds to the questions presented by the scenario. For example, the following scenario might be presented to a group of nurses on a medical unit:

*T*he physician writes new patient orders on a blue order form set. The nurse or unit secretary then transfers the written orders into the computer system. The person entering the orders initials the blue order form set to indicate that these orders were entered into the computer. A computer-generated order set is printed out and placed in the patient medical record. Prior to placing the computer order set in the patient chart, it is checked by the nurse to ensure accuracy and completeness. Audits of this process have shown that almost 30 percent of the time, the computer-generated order set is either inaccurate or incomplete. In 35 percent of the cases, the original orders on the blue order set have not been initialed. Additionally, 40 percent of the time, orders are not entered in a timely fashion, often exceeding 1 hour or more.

After the scenario is given or developed by the end-users, several prepared questions are asked by the interview team. For example, in the above scenario the following questions might be used:

- How must the current process be restructured so that error rates are reduced?
- What functions must be incorporated into the new computer system to ensure that error rates are minimal?
- What features must be included in the system to enhance the ease of data entry?

The scenario-based interview is more and more frequently becoming the interview method of choice. The technique provides a more realistic perspective of system requirements, features, and function by allowing end-users to respond to questions in the context of an existing situation. Thus, responses focus not only on system requirements but also on the current process and organizational environment. Many times, it is the way in which current work is performed that is the cause of work duplication, errors, and inefficiencies. Thus, before implementing any new or updated version of an information system, it is important to assess the work process for causes of inefficient or ineffective work output. In most instances, it is necessary to reengineer the work process before developing and implementing a new information system. Diagramming the flow of data from process to process in DFDs can be helpful in restructuring work processes.

In addition to interviewing, observation may be used by the development team to gather information about user requirements. Observation of users performing their tasks helps to identify (1) data flow among users and the information system; (2) number and classes of employees that rely on the information system; (3) the frequency and type of data that are being used; and (4) the environment in which the information system will operate.

Using the observation technique requires a great deal of skill and a mechanism for the structured recording of all observation results. To ensure that appropriate and useful information is gathered, the purpose of the observation should be well defined. A structured observation protocol should be developed that represents the purpose and salient elements to be collected and/or documented. For example, the purpose of the observation may be to determine how clinic registration personnel interact with incoming patients, identify what data are collected, and identify how these data are currently entered into the registration and appointment system. The ultimate reason for the observation may be to determine if new features can be added to the current information system in order to reduce duplication of work, lower error rates, or make data entry easier and more efficient. Because of the tedious nature of observation, the maximum period for any single observation period should not exceed 1 hour.

The observation technique is frequently used as an adjunct to the interview method. Observation allows the development team to confirm end-user statements about work processes, needed system features, or opinions about information systems currently in use. When face-to-face interviews and observation are used together, the development team has a higher probability of accurately documenting system requirements than when either of these methods is used alone.

Surveys and questionnaires are another method that can be used to gather data about system requirements. However, this technique is less reliable and usually does not provide an in-depth understanding of work processes, system requirements, and function. Questionnaires and surveys are best used when only gross or high-level information is being solicited to identify potential problems and/or areas for further examination. For example, questionnaires are frequently used to determine client satisfaction with an information system.

Adjuncts and Aids in Identifying User Requirements As we have already seen, the identification of user requirements can be aided by using JAD techniques. Like the iterative process of multiple interviews, JAD brings together a group of end-users and system developers for a concentrated period of time—perhaps hours or days—to determine system requirements. The JAD process is led by a facilitator who uses various data-gathering methods to extract facts and opinions from the group. These methods may include unstructured, semistructured, and structured questions, questionnaires, scenarios and case studies, brainstorming, and other nominal and consensus-building group techniques.

The benefit of using JAD is that the process is led by an outside facilitator who can coordinate and stimulate interaction between end-users and developers in a nonthreatening environment. This technique usually produces less biased results and facilitates group consensus and acceptance. In most system development processes there must be a give and take among various constituencies. Not every end-user group can expect to get 100 percent of what it wants or needs. The JAD process helps to facilitate an understanding among users and developers of the overriding priorities and needs required for the development of a system that is essentially, if not completely, satisfying. In addition, because of the concentrated time frame, JAD produces results in a significantly shorter time period than other methods.

A newer tool that can be used to facilitate JAD or other group processes is group decision support software (GDSS). GDSS is a software application that has been recently refined. It utilizes a network of workstations or laptop computers that are located together in conference or meeting rooms. The GDSS software incorporates word processing, text, and database manipulation, electronic worksheets, graphics, and communication capabilities.

With GDSS each participant is assigned a workstation or laptop computer during the meeting. A facilitator uses the GDSS as an adjunct for eliciting facts, opinions, and responses from the group. For example, the facilitator may administer a questionnaire to the group using the GDSS software and results can be automatically and immediately tabulated. The facilitator might also use the GDSS in a nominal group process such as brainstorming and direct participants to record their ideas on a certain subject. The group ideas can be quickly collected electronically and categorized in different ways by the facilitator or group. One major benefit of GDSS is the assurance of anonymity. Participants are able to more freely answer questions or provide opinions without the fear of criticism or stigmatism by other group members. GDSS significantly speeds up the development process and minimizes bias of response in most cases.

Documenting Data Flows, Uses, and Requirements

In order to keep track of all the information requirements for a system that have been gathered through interview and observation, the development team must use specific notations and a documentation process. This documentation process results in a graphical map about the data of the business and the various interactions or relationships among data. Like architects, engineers, or city planners who begin their planning for buildings, highways, or city layouts with sketches, the information systems development team also begins its development of an information system with maps or sketches about the flow of data. We have already seen a DFD example in Figure 5-7. This mapping begins the development of the data model.

The diagrams and resulting data model must be viewed as a tool for communication between the development team and the end-users. The data model specifies the data structure that represents the user's view of the data. The data model should be iteratively designed. It must be continually refined as more and more input is received from the end-user during interviews and/or observations. It is important that the data model diagrams be periodically reviewed by the end-user during the data modeling process to ensure accuracy of the data flows. The entire success of the application and database design is directly dependent on how accurately the data model describes the data flows, transactions, and user requirements.

Documenting Data Flows, Data Relationships, Uses, and Requirements As mentioned previously, specific data modeling tools and methods are used to assist in the development of the conceptual and external data models. As we have already seen, the final process is to pull the results of these documentation aids together in a package so that the proposed system to be developed is accurately represented. The entire package of diagrams, narratives, dictionaries or glossaries, and access patterns constitutes the enterprise data model. It is this documentation set that is given to the programming staff for physical database development.

Developing Data Model Diagrams

One of the functions of the health information manager in an increasingly computerized environment will be to assist with the development of data model diagrams for the enterprise. To demonstrate how a data model diagram might be produced, an emergency department scenario is used. As we have already seen, there are many methods for data modeling, such as the Chen ER method, the NIAM method, and the information engineering (IE) method. Because of its popularity, ease of use, and concept of top-down development, the James Martin method of information engineering is used to illustrate how a data model diagram may be developed.

Martin Information Engineering Style

The Martin IE method is based on the concept that when an enterprise manages its data and information processes efficiently, it can increase competitive advantage. An important part of efficient information management is the development of information systems to support the strategic thrusts of the enterprise.

Stages of the Martin IE Method

The Martin IE method consists of four stages. Each of these stages provides the foundation for the next stage:

1. *Information strategy planning:* This stage is concerned with how information systems can support the strategic goals of the organization and how technology can be used in new and creative ways to better improve the organization's competitive position. The example of Mt. Pleasant Hospital on page 109 demonstrates the idea of information strategy planning or ISP. At this stage, technological opportunities are identified to support critical success factors. In other words, an analysis is performed to determine how things are accomplished in the organization and how these functions might be improved with the use of information technology. ISP includes the basic functions of the enterprise and produces an overview entity-relationship diagram of the enterprise, its departments, and its functions.

2. *Business area analysis:* The identification of organizational critical success factors determines which business areas within the organization should be the top priority for analysis—that is, what business areas are most important to achieving the critical success factors of the organization; what are the processes and data necessary to make these units operate optimally; and how do the work processes and data interrelate? The overall data model developed in stage 1 is decomposed and a more specific data model of the business unit is developed.

3. *System design stage:* Various types of diagrams and charts are used during this stage. Among these are decomposition diagrams, data flow diagrams, data structure diagrams, as well as screen and report layouts. Frequently at this stage a prototype (or sample) of the system is developed. As we have learned, a prototype is usually not a functional system but an example of what the system will look like after it is fully developed. Prototyping is an iterative approach—that is, it goes through several stages. For example, if an emergency department system were being designed, an initial attempt would be made to build or design basic features of the system—perhaps input and output screens. The end-users of the system would review the first pass of the prototype and give input on necessary revisions and the addition of other features. The designers would then take this input and proceed to enhance the developing model. After incorporating these features and considering function, the prototype would again be reviewed by the end-users for additional input. This process continues over and over again, until an appropriate design is obtained.

4. *Construction of the system:* This stage includes the use of tools called code generators that generate computer code and the use of manual programming. A predominate aspect of this stage is the supervision and control of transforming logical and physical design specifications to implementation of the physical system design. Tasks include: developing an implementation schedule; monitoring and controlling implementation; creating application programs and data structures; and developing user and program documentation.

Enterprise-wide data model diagrams can be very large. In fact, if you consider how many entities there may be in an acute-care facility or clinic or home health agency, diagramming these entities and their relationships to each other may take several feet of paper. Since replicating a complete data model for an entire organization would be too large to do in this text, we will assume that an enterprise-wide data model has been built and we will focus on the development of a data model for a particular business area—the emergency department at Mt. Pleasant Hospital.

IE Concepts and Methods of Notation

There are several mechanical steps in the development of a data model diagram (Fleming and Von Halle, 1993). Each of these steps should be done in sequence to help in developing a robust model:

- Identifying the major entities
- Determining the relationships among the entities
- Determining the primary and alternate entity identifiers
- Determining all non–key attributes of the entities
- Validating the model through normalization
- Determining attribute business rules
- Integrating the model with other existing data models
- Analyzing the model for stability and growth

Identifying Primary Entities To develop a data model diagram, entities must be identified, their attributes must be defined, and relationships between entities must be described. An entity is anything about which data can be stored. In many instances, an entity is a noun. For example, an employee, patient, physician, bill, order, and invoice are all entities. For each of these entities, there are data to be stored. For the entity "patient," we would likely store data about the patient's name, sex, birthdate, address, and so on. In the notation style that we are using to build our data model, entities are represented as a rectangle with the name of the entity placed inside the rectangle. Figure 5-8 shows an entity in a rectangle.

Identifying Relationships among Entities The second step in developing a data model diagram is to determine the relationships among all the entities that have been identified. Relationships are usually verbs. For exam-

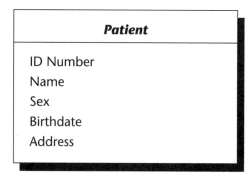

Figure 5-8.   Entity Representation

ple, a patient "has" a physician; a bill "is generated" for a patient; an employee "works" in a department. Relationships are represented in IE notation as lines between entities. There are, however, many different types of relations among data. For example, there are one-to-one relationships, one-to-many relationships, and many-to-many relationships. To accommodate these various relationships, various notational symbols are attached to the lines joining entities that have relations.

A one-to-one relationship is a relationship between two entities where for each occurrence of entity A there is one and only one occurrence of entity B. For example, for the entity "patient" and the entity "bed," there is a one-to-one relationship. In other words, one and only one patient can occupy bed 4B South, and similarly only one patient can occupy one bed at a time. Figure 5-9 shows a one-to-one relationship. Notice that the two entities "patient' and "bed" are represented by rectangles. A line joins each of these entities to show a relationship. Notice that a small bar is drawn across the line after the entity "patient" and before the entity "bed." This shows that each patient has only one bed and that each bed has only one patient.

A one-to-many relationship is an association between two entities where every occurrence of entity A is related to one or many occurrences of entity B, but every occurrence of entity B is related to only one occurrence of entity A. A good example of a one-to-many relationship is the relationship between medical orders and patients. In this case, every patient may have one or many orders. However, each individual order refers to only one patient. This relationship is depicted in Figure 5-10. The entity "patient" and the entity "medical order" are represented by rectangles. Note that a "crow's foot" is attached to the line before medical order

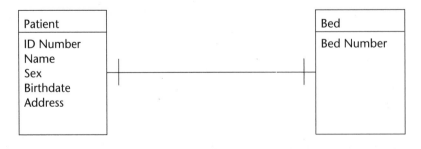

Figure 5-9.   One-to-One Relationship

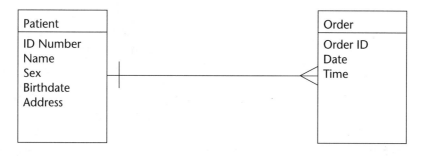

Figure 5-10. One-to-Many Relationship

to indicate that there may be one or many orders for each patient. Note also that a small bar is across the line after the entity "patient" to indicate that each individual order can only be associated with one patient.

A many-to-many relationship describes entities that have many relations in both directions. A good example is the relationship between the entity "surgeon" and the entity "patient." A surgeon can have many patients and a patient can have many surgeons. The many-to-many relationship is shown in Figure 5-11. Note that the entities "surgeon" and "patient" are represented by rectangles. Note also that crow's feet are attached to the line between both entities. This indicates the many-to-many relationship.

IE data model diagrams also indicate the minimum and maximum occurrences in a relationship. For example, there is a special notation that indicates that a relationship can have one, many, or no occurrences. This is

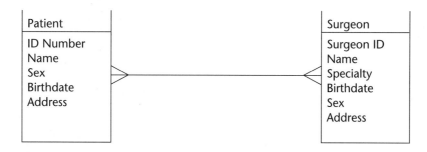

Figure 5-11. Many-to-Many Relationship

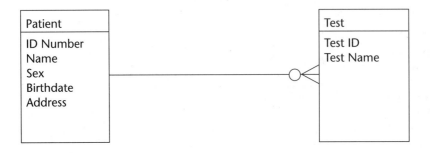

Figure 5-12. One–Many–None Relationship

represented by a small open circle placed before or after the crow's-foot notation. Figure 5-12 shows such a relationship.

In this example, the entity "patient" may have none, one, or many laboratory tests. The open circle preceding the crow's foot indicates the minimum occurrence (none) and the crow's foot indicates the maximum occurrence. Another notation is used to represent "one and only one" relationship. This is a double small bar across the relationship line. Figure 5-13 shows that a patient may have none, one, or many clinic visits, but each clinic visit can be associated with one and only one patient.

Determining Primary and Alternate Identifiers An attribute of an entity is a fact or piece of information about an entity. For example, attributes or facts about the entity "patient" would include the patient's first, middle, and last names, medical record number, street address, city, state, and zip code, sex, birthday, and so on. The specific occurrence of an entity can be identified by the values of its attributes. For example, Table 5-3 shows "patient." As

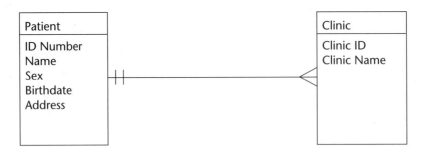

Figure 5-13. One and Only One Relationship

Table 5-3.   Example of Entity Patient

Medical Rec #	LNAME	FNAME	MINITIAL	BDATE	STREET ADDRESS	CITY	STATE	ZIP	SEX
893456	Brown	John	W	05-21-56	434 Oak	Sunshine	Ca	45678	Male
762345	Smith	Mary	J	03-21-60	8752 Palm	Sunshine	Ca	45678	Female
435678	Jones	Susan	J	01-03-72	7734 Citrus	Sunshine	Ca	45678	Female
256709	Castle	Joseph	E	04-08-66	7734 Citrus	Sunshine	Ca	45678	Male

you can see, John Brown can be distinguished from Mary Smith based on the values of the attributes of each of these entity occurrences. Usually not all attributes of an entity are required to identify a specific entity occurrence. For example, all the attributes listed in Table 5-3 would not be needed to identify specific occurrences of the patient entity. The attribute "medical record number" would be sufficient to identify a particular patient. An attribute (or a set of attributes) that uniquely identifies a particular occurrence of an entity is called an entity identifier or primary key.

In addition to having a primary key, an entity may also have alternate identifiers. These are attributes that are chosen as alternatives for identifying specific instances of an entity. For example, in Table 5-3, alternative identifiers, taken as a set, may include LNAME + BDATE + SEX. Alternative identifiers may also be called secondary keys.

Determining Non–Key Attributes After primary and secondary identifiers have been determined, non–key attributes are identified. Non–key attributes are descriptions that are usually associated with the entity. For example, in Table 5-3, the attributes STREET ADDRESS and CITY–STATE–ZIP ADDRESS are descriptions of the entity "patient."

Validating the Model through Normalization Once the data model has been initially developed, it is important to be sure that it truly represents the user's view. Normalization refers to how data items are grouped together. The process of normalization includes examining groups of data (in this case, attributes associated with an entity) to determine whether or not there are structural redundancies or inconsistencies due to assignment of an attribute with a wrong entity. An example of a misplaced attribute might be "lab test number" associated with the entity "patient." "Lab test number" is not usually descriptive of a patient, but would rather be more properly associated with an entity called "lab test."

Determining Alternate Business Rules Business rules govern the integrity of an entity. They determine certain properties or values that an attribute may have. For example, business rules determine the data type, length, format, uniqueness of values, allowable values, and default values of an attribute. The attribute "medical record number" would be governed by business rules that would determine its data type (numeric), length (seven characters), allowable values (0000001-9999999), default values (none), and so on.

Business rules also refer to triggering operations. These are rules that determine the correctness or incorrectness of data values. For example, the value of the attribute "discharge date" must be later than the value "admission date." Likewise, the value of the attribute "time and date medication ordered" must occur before the value of the attribute "time and date of medication administered."

Integrating the Model with Existing Models   In practice, data models for different business functions are developed in parallel or sequentially. Thus, when one model that represents a specific user group is developed, it must be integrated with other existing models. During consolidation, inconsistencies and overlaps will likely be detected and will need to be corrected. Consolidation of data models consists of comparing mappings and definitions of the models and the business conceptual schema. Inconsistencies may be discovered that include differences in names or application of business rules on attributes or relationships.

Analysis for Stability and Growth   The data model should also be analyzed in light of what future significant business changes may occur. These changes should be incorporated into the data model so that it will not need to be changed frequently and thus will remain stable while still allowing for growth.

A Sample Data Modeling Diagram Project

The following scenario is used as a foundation for illustrating the development of a data model diagram:

Mt. Pleasant Hospital has completed its strategic planning process. The organization identified five critical success factors (CSFs) that would need to be met if the organization wished to maintain a competitive advantage in the region:

1. Provide quality care.
2. Have efficient operations.
3. Develop good relationships with physicians.
4. Obtain optimal reimbursement and case mix.
5. Have a high perception of efficiency and service.

Once the CSFs for the organization were identified, various business areas were targeted as priority areas to ensure that the CSFs were being achieved. In addition, an enterprise-wide data model was developed that showed all the major entities within the enterprise and their relationship to each other. One of the top business areas that was targeted for evaluation was emergency department (ED) services. The ED was identified as a priority area because it was associated with all five of the CSFs: (1) there was room for improvement in the quality of care provided in the ED; (2) the operations of the ED were less than efficient; (3) attending physicians had complained on numerous occasions about ED inefficiencies; (4) data for patient bill generation were not satisfactory; and (5) patient satisfaction surveys had indicated that patients who used the ED were less than favorable about wait times. Because of these problems and their relationship to the organization's CSFs, the ED became a priority for business unit evaluation.

One of the first steps in evaluating the ED was to form a team of users, analysts, and database specialists. This team first identified the data flow in the department. In this case, a combination of techniques was used including face-to-face interviews and scenario analysis. Data flow was studied and resulted in the DFD that appears in Figure 5-14.

As Figure 5-14 demonstrates, the patient may arrive at the ED as either a walk-in or by some other way (i.e., helicopter, ambulance, etc.). When the patient arrives as a walk-in, the patient is registered and certain information is collected, such as name, chief complaint, address, birthdate, and so on. After the patient is registered, the patient is seen by the triage nurse. The nurse documents vital signs and other information and makes an assessment as to the urgency of the case. The patient is then put in a queue and when an examination room becomes available the patient is escorted to the room. There the patient sees a physician, who performs an examination, orders tests, writes prescriptions, makes a diagnosis, and makes a decision about patient disposition. At this point the patient may be retained in the ED for additional observation, admitted to the hospital, or discharged. If the patient is discharged, a discharge nurse provides the patient with discharge instructions and any other necessary materials, medications, or aids.

After the flow of work and data were studied, the development team wanted to collect some demographic information about the patient care and flow in the ED. For example, the team wanted to know:

- What are the most common diagnoses for patients seen in the ED?
- What is the average time it takes for a patient to receive diagnostic tests associated with specific chief complaints, such as chest pain, right lower abdominal pain, right upper quadrant abdominal pain, and so on?

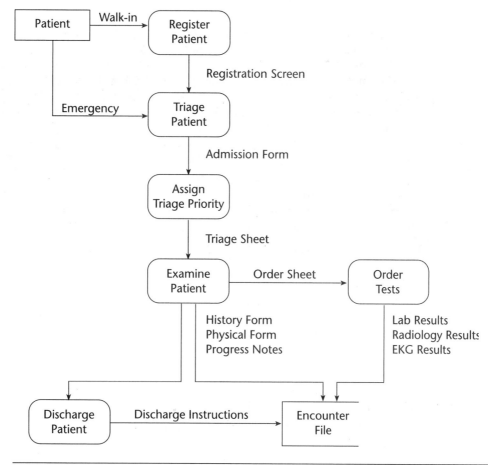

Figure 5-14. Data Flow of ED Process

- What are the predominant geographic areas from which the patients come?
- What is the distribution of services for patients with the same discharge diagnosis?
- What are the average wait times for a patient to receive diagnostic tests such as CBC, UA, chest x-ray, CT scan?
- Do physicians handle patients with similar demographics and the same chief complaint the same way? Are there differences in the standard of care?
- What are the predominant third-party payers?

It was discovered that these questions could not be answered because there was no information system, either manual or automated, that documented these data. The answers to these questions would serve as measures of efficiency and quality of care delivered by the ED. Therefore, it was not hard to realize that an information system was needed that would support the CSFs for helping to ensure and measure quality of care and better efficiency in the ED.

The next step in designing the information system needed for ED support was to review the enterprise data model diagram. Figure 5-15 is a sample of what an enterprise data model diagram might look like. This sample is overly simplified. If an actual model were included in this text, it would like take up several dozens of pages. However, Figure 5-15 provides a "flavor" for what an enterprise diagram might provide.

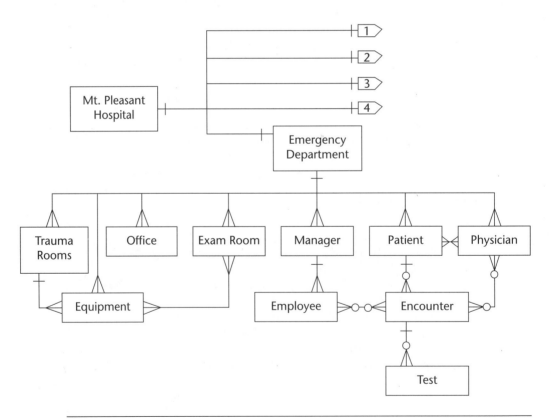

Figure 5-15. Enterprise Data Model: ED Conceptual Schema

In our sample enterprise data model diagram there is the entity "Mt. Pleasant Hospital" about which data can be stored. Within the hospital there are several departmental entities. This particular diagram shows the Emergency Department, but the diagram connector arrows numbered 1, 2, 3, and so on show that there are many more departmental entities within the hospital. The connector arrows indicate that these departments are explained on other pages of the model.

Figure 5-15 shows the ED as an entity with a one-to-one relationship with Mt. Pleasant Hospital. Because the ED is an entity, facts about it can be stored. For example, data stored about the ED would include its unique department number. Other entities related to the ED include office, equipment, exam room, trauma rooms, manager, employee, patient, physician, encounter, and test. Each of these entities has a relationship with the ED and also may have relations with other entities. For example, the ED has a one-to-many relationship with the entity "manager." In other words, the ED has many managers, but each manager is associated with only one ED. Looking further we see that there is a one-to-many relationship between the entity "manager" and the entity "employee." Each manager can have many employees but each employee will have only one manager.

In the scenario presented about the information system needs of Mt. Pleasant Hospital ED, we are primarily concerned with the entity "patient encounter" and its relationships with other entities. This is because the information system that we need to design to support the organizational CSFs is concerned primarily with supporting processes involving the efficiency and quality of the patient-care encounter. The shaded part in Figure 5-16 shows the entities of interest for developing the ED information system needed by Mt. Pleasant Hospital.

Figure 5-17 provides a schematic of the principal entities, their relationships, and attributes that represent the ED functions and will provide information to answer the questions for which the information system is to be designed. One of the most important steps in the development of a data model is to clearly understand the purposes for which the information system is being developed. In the example of Mt. Pleasant Hospital, the intent is to provide an information system that will support ED functions and answer questions related to efficiency and effectiveness of operations. Notice that none of the questions posed in the scenario relate to assisting with or evaluating the process of medical decision making. This is an important distinction. The way in which the data model is designed is directly dependent on the intended use of the information system. Notice that in the data model in Figure 5-17 there are few entities or attributes

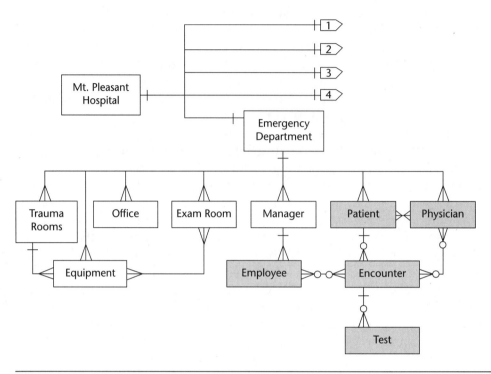

Figure 5-16.   Patient Encounter Relationships

associated with clinical information. If the intent of the information system for Mt. Pleasant would be to assist physicians in medical decision making, then a totally different data model would have to be designed. Entities related to clinical data and results of tests and treatments would need to be included in the data model. Frequently information systems fail because their purpose has not been clearly understood or defined.

In Figure 5-17, six entities are identified: patient, payer, encounter, professional staff, physician, test/treatment. Each of these entities is represented by a rectangle. The entity name is written at the top of the rectangle. For each of these entities, key and non–key attributes have been identified. Key attributes (unique identifiers) are underlined in the entity rectangle. Relationships among entities are represented using the standard notation that was described earlier in this chapter. Notice at the bottom of the diagram there are four domain tables. These tables represent files that contain values defining the constraints or business rules on the entity attributes.

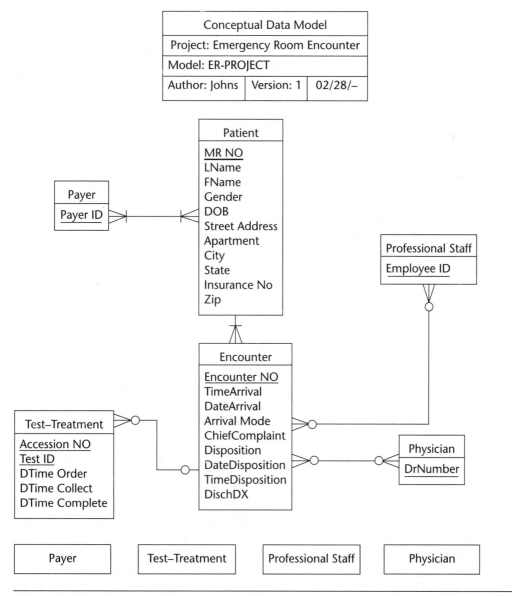

Figure 5-17. Conceptual ED Data Model

The data model can be interpreted in the following way:

Entity	Interpretation of Attributes and Relationships
Patient	The key attribute is medical record number. Other attributes include name, gender, birthdate, street address, apartment, city, state, insurance no., and zip. For each patient, there can be many encounters. For each patient, there can be many payers.
Payer	The key attribute for payer is payer ID. For each payer there can be many patients. There is a domain table for payer that defines the acceptable values of the payer ID attribute.
Encounter	The key attribute is encounter number. Other attributes include arrival date, arrival time, mode of arrival, chief complaint, disposition, discharge diagnosis, disposition date, and disposition time. For each encounter there is only one patient. For each encounter there may be none, one, or many professional staff. For each encounter there may be none, one, or many physicians. For each encounter there may be none, one, or many tests. For each encounter there may be none, one, or many treatments.
Professional Staff	The key attribute is staff ID number. There is a domain table associated with professional staff.
Physician	The key attribute is physician ID number. There is a domain table associated with physician.
Test/ Treatment	The key attribute is test/treatment ID number. Other attributes include time ordered, time collected, and time completed. For each test there is only one encounter. There is a domain table associated with test.

In addition to the data model diagram itself, other elements as we mentioned previously are part of the total data model package. These include: a list of data model entities; a list of all of the data attributes; a detailed description of each entity and a listing of all relationships.

Translation of the Conceptual Data Model to a Physical Data Model

Once the conceptual data model diagram has been developed, it can be translated into a physical database design. Specifics about the methodology for this translation are beyond the scope of this text and get into technical details with which the health information manager would normally not be involved. Briefly, however, the conceptual model is translated into a physical model through several steps including creating relations in the physical design and translating these into records, fields, and sets. Normally the relations in the physical design are the same as those in the conceptual design. After records, fields, and sets are created, the primary and secondary keys are implemented. CASE tools such as Sdesigner will translate the conceptual data model into a physical model. Figure 5-18 represents the physical database design for the ED example. Some of the concepts associated with physical database design are addressed in the next chapter.

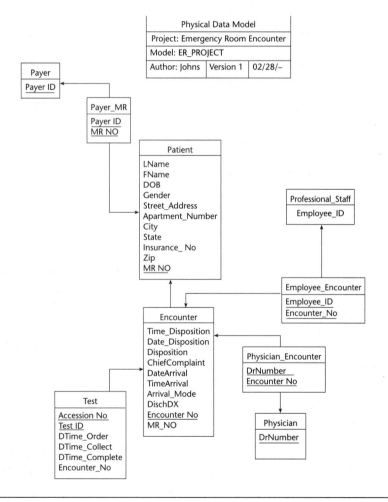

Figure 5-18.　Physical Data Model

Summary

- Data modeling is the process of determining the data that a business needs, identifying the relationships among these data, and graphically depicting these relationships as diagrams.

- Data modeling is a critical step in designing information systems that support the business functions and information needs of the organization. The data modeling process should be geared toward supporting the strategic thrusts of the organization so that a competitive advantage for the enterprise can be achieved.

- The health information manager should assume a prominent role between end-users and database designers, serving as a liaison in helping to identify end-user information requirements and ensuring that the purposes for which the information system are being developed are clearly articulated and understood.

- There are three types of data models: conceptual, external, and internal models. The conceptual model defines the database requirements of the entire enterprise. The external model is the view of the data by a specific group of users. The internal model depicts how the data are physically represented in the database.

- The contents of a conceptual data model include diagrams, glossaries, narratives, and access patterns.

- Entities, attributes, and relationships among entities are depicted in data model diagrams.

- Computer-assisted software engineering (CASE) tools are used to assist the designer in the development of data models.

- The most popular styles used for development of data model diagrams include the Chen entity-relationship (ER) method, the information engineering (IE) style, and the Nijssen information analysis methodology (NIAM).

Review Questions

1. Why is it important to develop a conceptual enterprise data model?
2. Explain how you would go about organizing a data model development effort.

3. Why would you want to use CASE tools in the data model development process?

4. Describe the contents of a conceptual data model. Why is each item important to the data modeling process?

5. What roles should the health information manager assume in the data modeling process?

Enrichment Activities

1. Select a business unit within a health-care enterprise (i.e., pharmacy, admitting, central supply, utilization management, quality improvement) and conduct a requirements interview with three or four employees. Conduct the interview using an interview protocol or scenarios. From the interview develop a draft of an external data model diagram. Be sure to use a standard notation such as ER or IE style.

2. Review an enterprise or business unit data model with a health-care information systems director. What type of CASE tools were used in the development effort? Why were these specific tools chosen over other tools? What type of notation did the development team use? What were the benefits to the team in developing the conceptual or external model?

References

Brown, Robert (1993). "Data modeling methodologies—contrasts in style. In Barbara Von Halle and David Kull (eds.), *Handbook of data management*. Boston, MA: Auderbach Publications.

Fleming, Candace C. and Von Halle, Barbara (1993). Building a data model. In Barbara Von Halle and David Kull (eds.), *Handbook of data management*. Boston, MA: Auderbach Publications.

Gause, Donald C., and Weinberg, Gerald M. (1989). *Exploring requirements quality before design*. New York: Dorset House Publishing.

Perry, W. E. (1993). Assessing the value of CASE technology. In P.C. Tinnirello (ed.), *Handbook of systems management development and support 1993–94 yearbook*. Boston: Auderback Publications.

Chapter 6

Database Management Concepts

Learning Objectives

After completing this chapter, the learner should be able to:

1. Discuss the differences between conceptual and physical data models
2. Differentiate between files, records, and fields.
3. Differentiate between file and database processing environments.
4. Differentiate between database models including relational, network, hierarchical, and object-oriented models.
5. Define the functions of a database management system (DBMS).
6. Describe the roles of a data administrator (DA).
7. Describe the Request for Proposal (RFP) document and process.

Key Terms

Authorization Rules
Concurrent Processing Control
Data Administrator
Data Dictionary
Data Integrity

Data Manipulation Languages

Data Redundancy

Database

Database Administrator

Database Management Systems

Encryption

Field

File

File Processing

Record

Recovery

Request for Proposal

Introduction

Chapter 5 introduces concepts and principles associated with data modeling. One of the important roles for the health information manager to assume is that of liaison between users and systems developers. In this role the health information manager has several functions, one of which is facilitating the development of the conceptual data model. According to the model of professional practice presented in Chapter 1, the health information manager assumes additional roles associated with database administration. In order to perform these functions, it is essential that the health information manager have a fundamental knowledge of the development and management of database systems and how physical data models are derived from conceptual data models.

As we saw, the conceptual data model is the precursor to development of the internal data model and physical databases. The conceptual data model lays the foundation for database development by identifying important entities, their attributes, and the relationships among entities. This groundwork provides an essential understanding of the information needs required to support the business processes of the organization.

The conceptual data model is transformed into a physical model by a sequence of steps. CASE tools can be used to transform the conceptual model into a physical or internal data model. Figure 6-1 shows the concep-

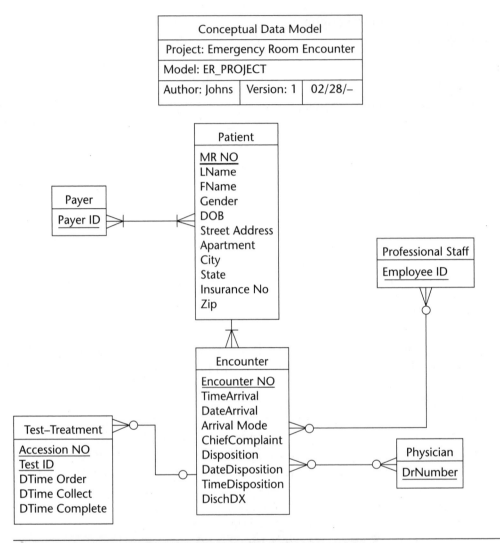

Figure 6-1.   Conceptual Data Model

tual data model and Figure 6-2 the relational physical data model of the emergency department (ED) presented in Chapter 5. The conceptual model was transformed using a CASE tool called Sdesigner. Notice the differences between the two models. The conceptual data model represents the user's view of how the data should be organized and displayed.

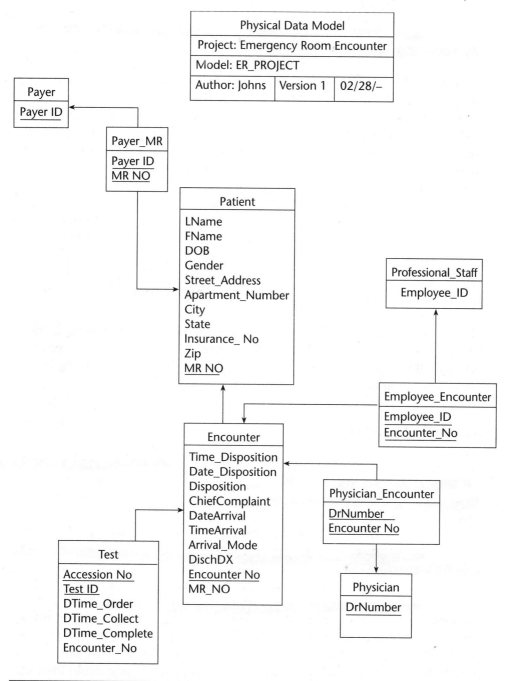

Figure 6-2. Physical Data Model

The physical data model, however, represents how the data are physically stored in database files.

In today's information-intensive health-care environment it is essential to not only know what an organization's information needs are but also to design and develop automated systems that best support those needs. Databases and their associated database management systems (DBMS) are essential components in any enterprise information architecture. As the uses of these systems expand and, in fact, are basic components in the development of the computer-based patient record (CPR), new roles in the administration of data are emerging for the health information manager. The purpose of this chapter is to introduce the learner to basic concepts associated with databases and their management and to present an overview of the roles that the health information manager can assume.

Database and Database Management Concepts

This section introduces basic concepts associated with databases, database management systems (DBMS), and physical data models. The intent is to explain these concepts using the emergency department example presented in Chapter 5.

Files, Records, and Fields

The most fundamental concepts associated with the conceptual data model are entities, attributes, and relationships. As we have previously learned, an entity is a person, location, thing, or concept about which data can be collected and stored. For example, common entities encountered in the health-care environment include patient, physician, encounter, and employee. An attribute describes an entity and is sometimes thought of as the property of an entity. As we have previously seen, common attributes of the entity "patient" include name, gender, birthdate, and medical record number. Relationships are associations between entities. As Chapter 5 demonstrates, relationships may be one-to-one, one-to-many, or many-to-many. A logical question to ask in studying the transformation from a conceptual data model to an internal physical data model is "How are entities, attributes, and relationships of the conceptual model handled in the database environment?"

In the physical database environment, the critical concepts are **field, record,** and **file.** If you have previously taken a computer course, you know that the smallest piece of datum that can be stored is a bit. A collection of bits make up a character. For example, a character can be alphabetical (a, b, c, d), numeric (1, 2, 3, 4), or special (#, @, &). A character or a collection of characters make up a field. The designation "M" for male or "F" for female would make up the field "sex"; or the collection of characters 03-21-48 would make up the field "birthdate." A collection of fields represents a record. "Medical record number," "name," "sex," and "birthdate" would constitute a record. A collection of records (or occurrences of a record) constitute a file. Figure 6-3 displays the concepts of file, record, and fields. Note that in Figure 6-3 the file is called "Patient," the columns represent fields or data elements, and the rows represent records.

You might have already ascertained that for each entity in the conceptual model there is a file in the physical database. For example, look at Figure 6-1. Notice that in the conceptual model there is an entity called "patient." Notice that in the physical model (Figure 6-2) there is also an entity called "patient." As you might expect, attributes in the conceptual model are analogous to fields in the physical model. Again, looking at Figure 6-1, note that the attributes of the entity "patient" all appear in the physical model as fields in the file "Patient."

The conceptual model also describes relationships between entities. These same relationships must be translated to the physical model, which is accomplished by placing the key attribute (unique identifier) of one entity as a field in the entity with which it has a relation. The placement of

Patient File

Med Rec No	Lname	Fname	MidInitial	Sex	Birthdate
445678	Hunt	Denise	M	F	04-21-78
567890	Prentice	Dorothy	A	F	08-15-29
754231	O'Rafferty	Jennifer	A	F	03-12-86
987321	Mohle	Robert	E	M	12-16-61
889012	Martin	Paula	R	F	04-08-35
776324	Pilon	Denis	N	M	02-14-17

Figure 6-3.   Representation of a File Structure

this key identifier in another entity is sometimes referred to as a foreign key. For example, the key attribute in the entity "patient" is "medical record number." Notice also that the medical record number is the key field in the file "Patient." In looking at Figure 6-2, we can see that in the physical model the field "medical record number" is added as a field in the "Encounter" file. Remember that in the conceptual data model the relationship between the entity "patient" and the entity "encounter" is a one-to-many relationship. By placing the unique identifier "medical record number" as a foreign key in the file "Encounter," this one-to-many relationship is represented.

Representing the relationships among entities is important for data retrieval purposes. For example, say we wanted to retrieve data for all the encounters a specific patient had during 1995. We would use the value of the patient's medical record number and search through all the records in the "Encounter" file. Because the value of the field "medical record number" is present in the file "Encounter," all the records pertaining to that patient would be retrieved. However, if the foreign key "medical record number" had not been included in the file "Encounter," there would be no easy way of retrieving data for this query. Likewise, using this method we would be able to find out detailed information about patients who had certain types of encounters. For example, say we wanted a list of all patients who had been seen in the emergency department with a chief complaint of chest pain. Because the foreign key "medical record number" has been included as a field in the record "encounter," the computer could search the "Encounter" file for the chief complaint of chest pain and could search the "Patient" file for the patient name using the value in the "medical record number" field. In a many-to-many relationship, such as that existing between the entities "physician" and "encounter," the key attributes or fields of each entity are included as a foreign key in the other entity. Note how this task is accomplished in the physical model depicted in Figure 6-2.

File versus Database Processing

The database processing environment is much different from the typical file processing arena. Prior to the development of database systems, **file processing** was the typical processing environment. Even today there are many health-care facilities still operating in a file environment.

In the usual file processing environment, each user area has its own files. For example, health information management, dietary, business office, quality management, utilization management, and physician credentialing may have their own group of files and application programs that access these files. Figure 6-4 displays part of the files for some of these departments.

One of the first problems that you notice with such a collection of files is data duplication. Notice that all the files contain fields for the patient's birthdate and admit date. The diagnostic and utilization management files duplicate several fields including admit date, discharge date, sex, and diagnostic code. This duplication of data fields is called **data redundancy.**

There are several problems associated with data redundancy. First, it consumes a lot of space. However, poor space utilization is not necessarily the most important problem. Update of the files is also problematic. When the patient's address changes, it must be updated in both the Patient and the Business Office files. If the patient is transferred from one unit or bed to another, then the bed information in the Dietary and Utilization Management files must be updated. Coordination and communication for update of separate files is difficult and can consume an enormous amount of employee time.

Two of the biggest problems associated with data redundancy, however, are poor data integrity and difficult data retrieval. **Data integrity** usually refers to the consistency of data. Looking at the Patient, Diagnostic, and Utilization Management files reveals that the birthdate for Tara Jones is different in each file. Notice also that the final diagnosis codes in the Business and Diagnostic files do not agree for Tara Jones. Poor data integrity is often a result of storing and processing data in a file environment.

Data retrieval is also a significant problem in a file environment. For example, say a facility wants to analyze data to determine if there is a difference in the patient severity index among payers. These data might be useful in developing managed-care contracts with various payers. In order to retrieve these data using the files in Figure 6-4 , at least two and maybe three files would have to be queried—these include the Business Office, Diagnostic, and Utilization Management Files. This process can be extremely time-consuming and the data retrieved may not be consistent. For instance, look at the admit dates for Tara Jones in the Utilization Management and Diagnostic files. Because these codes do not agree (poor data

Patient File

Pt Number	Pt Name	Address	Birthdate	Sex	Admit Date	Discharge Date
887456	John Smith	Anytown	3-21-50	M	7-7-96	7-21-96
798011	Tara Jones	Anytown	5-25-51	F	7-9-96	8-1-96

Diagnostic File

Pt Number	Admit Date	Discharge Date	Sex	Birthdate	Dx Code	Physician No
887456	7-7-96	7-21-96	M	3-20-50	250.01	87990
798011	7-9-96	8-1-96	F	5-25-51	410.01	45600

Dietary File

Pt Name	Admit Date	Sex	Birthdate	Room No	Diet Code	Bed #	Diet Description
John Smith	7-7-96	M	3-21-50	405West	6789	1	N/A
Tara Jones	7-9-96	F	5-25-96	215East	0990	2	N/A

Business Office File

Acct #	Pt Name	Admit Date	Discharge Date	Birthdate	Payer No	Address	Dx Code
7654	John Smith	7-7-96	7-21-96	3-20-50	8790	Anytown	250.01
0978	Tara Jones	7-9-96	8-1-96	5-25-51	8790	Anytown	410.09

Utilization Management File

Pt Number	Birthdate	Admit Date	Discharge Date	Dx Code	Critical Path #	Bed #	Sex
887456	3-21-55	7-7-96	7-21-96	250.00	567	1	M
798011	5-25-51	7-11-96	8-1-96	410.01	123	2	F

Figure 6-4. File Processing Environment

integrity), the data analyst is faced with the problem of determining which one is correct.

One mechanism to overcome problems caused by data redundancy is to build a system that can store data about more than one entity and show relationships among entities. The idea of a database is fairly uncomplicated. Instead of storing information about only one entity as in the file processing environment, information can be stored about multiple entities and the relationships among these entities. Thus, a **database** is a structure that allows for the storage of data about multiple entities and the relationships among these entities. Figure 6-5 shows how a database might be constructed that stores data about multiple entities.

Notice that in Figure 6-5 duplication of data among files is reduced. Because data about multiple entities and their relationships are stored together, there is less duplication of data. For example, the diagnosis, business, dietary, and utilization management files (tables) have now been reduced. Data specific to the patient and to the encounter are stored in the Patient and Encounter tables. Notice that data retrieval can be accomplished across the various files (tables) because relationships among the entities have been established through the use of key identifiers and foreign keys. As an example, the Business Office file now contains the foreign key encounter number that relates it to the Encounter table. Because of this relationship, information about the encounter, such as admit date and discharge date does not need to be duplicated in the Business Office table but can be stored in one place but accessed through foreign keys by multiple files. Taking the Patient table and Business table we could easily produce a listing of patient names and addresses with insurance coverage provided by payer code 200.

A database is virtually useless unless the data can be used by application programs and updated and queried by the user. The task of managing the database so that these functions can be accomplished is very complex. Therefore, specific software programs exist that are called **database management systems** (DBMS) to facilitate these functions. A DBMS allows users to interact with the database and also performs all the underlying manipulations to maintain the database. For example, the DBMS provides the mechanisms that allow users to add, update, delete, and retrieve data. Using the query, "Provide a listing of patient names and addresses with insurance coverage by payer 200" as an example, the DBMS would locate and access the appropriate files, records, and fields to answer the query. This function releases the user from having to know what files contain the needed information or how these files are structured or indexed.

Patient Table

Pt Number	Pt Name	Address	Birthdate	Sex
887456	John Smith	Anytown	3-21-50	M
798011	Tara Jones	Anytown	5-25-51	F

Encounter Table

Encounter No	Admit Date	Discharge Date	Room #	Bed #	Pt Number
12345678	7-7-96	7-21-96			887456
12345679	7-9-96	8-1-96			798011

Diagnostic Table

Dx Code	Encounter No	MD No
250.01	887456	87990
410.01	798011	

Dietary Table

Diet Code	Diet Description	Encounter No
6789	N/A	12345678
0978	N/A	12345679

Business Office Table

Payer No	Encounter No	Acct No
8790	12345678	7654
8790	12345679	0978

Utilization Management Table

Critical Path#	Encounter #
567	12345678
123	12345679

Figure 6-5. Database Environment

A major advantage of a DBMS is that it provides each user or user group with its own view of the database. Separating the database into multiple, simpler views makes manipulation of the database easier for the user as well as provides a mechanism for data security. A user view (part of the database) is often referred to as a *subschema* and the entire database is often called a *schema*.

User views or subschemas are created by the database administrator. In basic terms, the user view is a pseudofile that consists of data fields to which a user may have access. Data do not actually exist in this file, but are derived from the actual database files whenever the user attempts to access the view. Examine the database example in Figure 6-5. There are six files contained in the database. However, not all users need access to all of these data. The dietary department, for instance, would not need access to any of the data fields in the Business or Utilization files. The data fields most useful to a user in the dietary department would probably include diet code, room/bed number, patient number, patient name, birthdate, and diagnosis description. Therefore, these data fields would compose the subschema or user view for a dietary employee.

User views or subschemas have several benefits. The database is much simpler for the user. Also through the use of subschemas the database administrator can control access to data fields on a need-to-know basis. Thus, employees have access to only those data items that are essential to perform their work tasks. Another benefit of user views is that they are independent of the physical structure of the database files—that is, the physical structure of the database may be changed, but as long as no data fields are removed to which a user needs access, none of the user application programs need to be changed.

In addition to the features already discussed, a DBMS performs many other functions such as providing concurrency, security, and integrity controls. These tasks are explained in detail later in this chapter.

Database Structure Models

A DBMS can use one of several approaches to store and manipulate data. A basic knowledge of these methods is useful to the health information manager in understanding DBMS operation. These methods encompass the physical data model and include four approaches: relational, network, hierarchical, and object-oriented models. Regardless of the approach used, each data model has two components: structure and operations. System structure is the way users perceive the system to be constructed or the way data are organized. Operations refers to the facilities given to users to manipulate the data within the database. It is not the intent of this chapter to discuss in detail technical aspects of these approaches, but rather to present an introduction and overview of these models as well as the relative strengths and weaknesses of each one.

Relational Model

The relational database model was first proposed in 1970 (Codd, 1970). During the 1970s, the relational model was studied and was the subject of many research efforts. Prototype systems were developed during this time and in the 1980s commercial relational database systems started to appear both in the mainframe and microcomputer environments.

A relational data model is perceived by the user to consist of a collection of tables. Figure 6-6 presents a user's view of a relational database model for the emergency department example described in Chapter 5. Notice that the data are arranged in tables that have columns and rows. Formally these tables are called *relations*. Entities, attributes, and entity relationships are implemented in the tables. In the relational model each entity gets a table of its own. As we can see in Figure 6-6, there is a table for each of the emergency department entities. The attributes of the entity become columns in the table. The attributes for each entity are represented as columns. Relationships among entities are represented by common columns. For example, in our conceptual data model of the emergency department (Figure 6-1), the entity "patient" was a one-to-many relationship with the entity "patient encounter." To represent this relationship in the relational model, the unique identifier "medical record number" from the "patient" table is added as a column (foreign key) in the "encounter" table. With this type of structure we can answer specific queries about patients and encounters. For instance, we can determine how many encounters a patient has had and we can use this column to determine what patient was treated during the encounter.

There are many conventions or rules that must be met in designing a relational database model. Looking at Figure 6-6, notice that each column has a unique name and entries within that column match the column name. In other words, in the column "medical record number" we would

Payer File

Payer ID

Patient File

MR #	**Name**	**Sex**	**Birthdate**	**Street**	**City**	**State**	**Zip**

Encounter File

Date	**Arrival Time**	**Mode of Arrival**	**Chief Complaint**	**Disposition**	**Discharge Date**	**Discharge Time**	**Dx Code**	**MR #**

Professional Staff File   *Physician File*   *Test/Treatment File*

Employee ID	**Encounter #**	**Physician ID**	**Encounter #**	**Test #**	**Time Ordered**	**Time Completed**	**Encounter #**

Domain Tables: Professional Staff Table
                 Payer Table
                 Test/Treatment Names
                 Physician Table

Figure 6-6.   Emergency Department Relational Database

expect to see a six-digit number that is in fact a medical record number. Another rule in the relational model is that all rows must be unique—that is, no two rows can have exactly the same data.

A final constraint in designing a relational database model is that multiple entries (repeating groups) for one position are not allowed—that is, each position is restricted to one entry. Figure 6-7 shows a table for an ED encounter that violates the repeating group convention. Notice that for patient 127378 there are three entries in the Final Diagnosis column. There

Patient Number	Physician #	Final Diagnosis #	Admit Date	Discharge Date
127377	4567	210.76	8/15/95	8/21/95
127378	8892	250.01	8/10/95	8/30/95
		110.37		
		410.7		
233898	7345	786.92	8/1/85	8/5/95

Figure 6-7. Example of Repeating Groups

are various way of correcting the problem of repeating groups. One way is to create another table (entity) for final diagnosis that will have a one-to-many relationship with the entity "ED encounter."

Sometimes the terminology associated with relational database models is confusing. When the relational model was first proposed, the terms *relation, tuple,* and *attribute* were used to describe the relational model. The table itself, as we mentioned before, is referred to as a *relation.* To be technically correct, each row in the table is referred to as a *tuple* and each column is referred to as an *attribute.* Since the 1970s, alternate language has developed to describe these concepts. Today there are two commonly used alternatives to the technical or formal terms. A comparison of these terms is provided below. The most commonly used terminology today is Alternative One.

Formal Terms	Alternative One	Alternative Two
Relation	Table	File
Tuple	Row	Record
Attribute	Column	Field

The relational database model has several advantages over the hierarchical, network, and object-oriented models that are discussed later. An important advantage of the relational database model is that it is generally easier for end-users to use than other models. A variety of mechanisms exist to assist end-users in querying the database. These mechanisms are referred to as **data manipulation languages** (DML). Several DML approaches exist including structured query language (SQL) and query by example (QBE). SQL is the most popular DML and most relational DBMS use a version of SQL or a DML that is similar to it.

Another advantage of the relational database model is that it maintains data independence—that is, changes can be made in the database structure without having to make changes in the programs that access the database. Obviously this has important implications in regard to human resources required to update many programs every time a change is made in the physical database structure. The relational model promotes a much higher degree of data independence than, say, the hierarchical and network models.

While the relational model has several advantages over the other database models, it also has some drawbacks. The chief disadvantage concerns efficiency. Critics of the relational model claim that it is not as efficient as some hierarchical or network models. Basically the computer must do more work to retrieve and store data in a relational database environment. Therefore, the relational model may not be appropriate for developing very large-scale application programs. Proponents of the relational model, however, counter that the gap between the relational model and other models is quickly closing and that relational models can be as efficient as many hierarchical and network models.

Network Model

The network database model was originally developed in the late 1960s. The most prominent system development effort, called Integrated Data Store or IDS, was led by Charles Bachman at General Electric. This system was the precursor to the common network model approach called CODASYL. Most network systems today follow the CODASYL approach.

Just like the relational model, the network model represents entities, their attributes, and relationships among entities within its structure. The network model represents these concepts in a different way than the relational model. In the network model, entities are referred to as record types, attributes are referred to as fields within a record type, and relationships are explicitly defined in terms of sets. Figure 6-8 is a representation of three of the emergency department entities and their relationships in a network model. The rectangles represent the record types (entities) in the database. The arrows represent the one-to-many relationships among entities. The arrow goes from the "one" part to the "many" part. Therefore, in

Figure 6-8 one patient has many encounters but one encounter can have only one patient; one encounter has many tests but one test can have only one encounter. The relationship between patient and encounter is called a set. Likewise, the relationship between encounter and tests is called a set. Sets are given names. The set from patient to encounter is called "Has" because each patient has an encounter. The set from encounter to tests is called "Composed of" because each encounter is composed of tests. There is specific terminology that is also used to describe these relationships. The record type "patient" is referred to as the "owner" of the record type "encounter" and "encounter" is referred to as a "member" of "Patient."

Figure 6-8 represents only the emergency department entities with a one-to-many relationship. You might be wondering how many-to-many

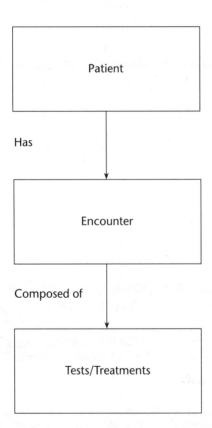

Figure 6-8. Network Database Model

relationships are handled in a network model. Within the network model, and more specifically the CODASYL model, there is no facility for handling many-to-many relationships. (The CODASYL model is used interchangeably with the concept of a network model.) Thus, these types of relationships have to be represented through another record type called a *link record.* The mechanics of implementing the link record type are not important, however, for our discussion here.

The network model database is manipulated essentially by following the arrows. Arrows can be followed in either direction. For example, if we follow the arrow from "patient" to "encounter," we will retrieve all the encounters that a particular patient has had in the emergency department. If we follow the arrow in the reverse direction from "encounter" to "patient," we will retrieve information about the single patient who was the object of a given emergency department encounter.

Figure 6-9 provides a diagram to illustrate how data are queried or manipulated in a network database model. We can see that there are three occurrences of the record type "patient," six occurrences of the record type "encounter," and ten occurrences of the record type "test." Thus, patient 1 has three encounters and encounter 1 is composed of three tests. If we would want to know how many encounters patient 1 had, we would ask the DBMS to find patient 1. After patient 1 was found, we would repeatedly ask the DBMS to find the next encounter among the collection of encounters for patient 1 until the last encounter had been located. The first time we made the request, we would obtain encounter 1; the second time we made the request we would obtain encounter 2; the next time we made the request we would obtain encounter 3; the fourth time we made the request the DBMS would indicate that there were no more encounters to be found.

Queries to the database are not always fulfilled by transversing the network from owner to member. Sometimes it is necessary to transverse the database in the opposite direction. For example, suppose we wanted to know who was treated during encounter 1. To answer this query we would ask the DBMS to find encounter 1. We would then ask the DBMS to find the owner of encounter 1. The owner is a single patient in this case.

Network models are very efficient and are able to handle large databases with a lot of activity. Network systems also have better facilities for ensuring data integrity. For example, information about an encounter could not be added to a network database before information about a patient was entered. This type of check ensures that there is not incomplete or "orphaned" data in the database.

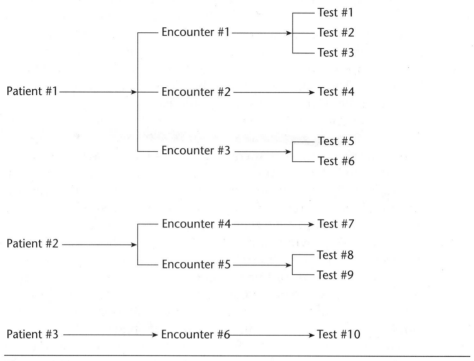

Figure 6-9.   Representation of Network Query

Network systems, however, have several disadvantages. As opposed to the relational model, it is not as easy for users to manipulate data in the network approach. In order to retrieve the desired information out of a network system, the user needs to know what path (arrows) to follow. Thus, an actual knowledge of the underlying database structure is needed to follow the right path to satisfy a given query. Second, it is more difficult to make changes in the network model than in a relational system. As you will recall, changes can be made in a relational system without necessarily causing changes in application programs. However, this is not the case in the network method. When changes in a database using a network model are made, changes are also required in all the programs that access that part of the database that has been changed.

Hierarchical Model

A hierarchical model is perceived by a user to be composed of a hierarchy or trees. A hierarchical model is a special case of a network model. Basically the model is a network with an added restriction—no record type (entity) can have more than one arrow entering it, although it may have more than one arrow leaving it. In addition to this restriction, the terminology between the two methods differs as well. For example, in the network model, relationships among entities are referred to as sets and these sets are given names. There is no analogous naming of relationships in the hierarchical approach. Other terminology varies as well. For example, in network models, the "one" end of a relationship is referred to as the "owner" and the "many" end of a relationship is referred to as a "member." In the hierarchical model, the "one" end of the relationship is called a "parent" and the "many" end of the relationship is called a "child." Although different strategies are employed to store and manipulate the data, the navigation of a hierarchical model is similar to that described for a network model.

Hierarchical systems provide advantages over the relational model similar to those of the network model. Basically the advantages are efficiency and data integrity protection. The disadvantages of the network model apply to the hierarchical model as well, including issues relating to changes in the underlying data structure that also require changes in affected application programs and cumbersome methods of data manipulation for end-users.

Object-Oriented Models

There has been a great deal interest in the development of an object-oriented approach to system design and development. There are object-oriented programming languages as well as object-oriented databases. An object-oriented database is perceived by the user to be a collection of objects. Each object essentially represents an entity. However, in addition to the attributes being stored within the object, an object can store other objects as well. An object can also include actions that can be taken on that object. For example, actions that might be taken on a "patient" object (entity) may include add patient, change address, and change payer. Actions that can be taken on an object can also be part of the data definition and used whenever they are needed. In contrast, a non-object-oriented system implements actions as part of its data manipulation process and the actions appear in the programs that update or change the database.

A big advantage of the object-oriented approach is that in addition to containing text and numbers, an object can also contain complex data types such as pictures, graphics, and sound. This is of particular interest in the health-care field where a lot of clinical data are represented as pictures, graphs, x-rays, and so on.

Database Management System Functions

As we have seen, a database environment has several advantages over a traditional file processing environment. First, a database approach to data storage and retrieval reduces data redundancy. Reducing data redundancy reduces the space it takes to store data. It also reduces the amount of human resources and time it takes to update data. As we saw in our examples of the file processing environment, when data are updated they must be changed in every single file throughout the organization that needs that particular information update. This update process can consume enormous amounts of personnel time. Another benefit to reducing data redundancy is that there is a better chance for improving data integrity. As we saw in our file processing example in the beginning of this chapter, data located in different independent files are frequently inconsistent. Many times organizations retrieve the "same" data from different files only to find that the data do not say the same thing. There is also a problem with inconsistent naming and definition of data items. For example, one departmental file may label the patient medical record number as "patient number" and another departmental file may call the same number "patient identifier." Although this inconsistency may not seem important on the surface, it has serious implications when there are attempts to retrieve the same data from different files.

Another important advantage of a database approach is that the physical structure of the data are independent of the enterprise schema and user subschemas or views. Thus, changes can be made in the physical structure of the database without affecting the user view of the data (i.e., how the user uses the data). It also means that application programs need not be rewritten every time there is a change in the physical structure of the database. As we have already learned, this is particularly true with the relational model approach to database design.

While the database approach to the storage and retrieval of data has several advantages, the management of the database approach is very complex. In order to manage this complicated system, a software tool was developed called a database management system. In basic terms, the DBMS software can be thought of as a "middle man" that facilitates interface of users with the physical database. When a query is made to the database, it is the DBMS that determines what data should be accessed, by whom the data can be accessed, and what data can be released. When data need to be added, changed, or deleted in the database, it is the DBMS that ensures that the correct sequence of events occurs to perform the required function.

There are many different DBMS software packages available. Regardless of the vendor or approach, all of these systems essentially provide:

1. Update and storage of data
2. A catalog (data dictionary) of descriptions of the data
3. A natural user interface
4. Transaction support
5. Utilities to ensure data integrity
6. Concurrent processing controls
7. Recovery services
8. Authorization controls (security)

An important part of the health information manager's role is to understand what functions the DBMS should provide. Each of these functions is discussed in more detail below.

Storing, Retrieving, and Updating Functions

How does a DBMS handle the operations for storage, retrieval, and update of data? While there are many technical procedures that are followed to perform these functions, our concern is with an overview of the process. As we know, data reside on disk in a physical database. The DBMS must access this physical database in order to retrieve, store, or update data. Remember that the DBMS acts as a "middle man" between the physical database and the user and application programs. Acting in its role as middle man, the DBMS receives a request from an admitting clerk using an application program to update information on patient John Smith #224567. Using various techniques, the DBMS identifies the record to be updated and instructs the operating system to read the record. The record is loaded into the computer buffers and the DBMS determines what data are required to fulfill the original user request. The DBMS then authorizes transfer of the data from system buffers back to the application program from where the request originated. The required data are now located in the user work area, and the user can now perform the necessary operations to update the record. Once the changes have been made by the user, the application program automatically sends an instruction to the DBMS to write back the updated record. Although this process is complicated, it virtually goes unnoticed by the user—that is, the user does not have to be concerned with all the algorithms and procedures that are necessary to ensure that the operations are performed. Instead, all the user does is ask the application program to update a record. In this instance, the admitting clerk probably selects an update feature on the admitting system. This is usually performed by selecting a choice on a menu, issuing a simple command, or if using a graphical user interface, selecting an icon to carry out the task. All the operations to locate the record, retrieve it, and bring it into the user work area are transparent to the user. All the user sees on the screen is the current patient information and the utilities to change that data.

Data Dictionary

One of the important functions of a DBMS is to catalog all the information about the database itself. The following information is usually provided in the **data dictionary** (DD).

- The names of records and fields contained in the database
- Characteristics about the fields such as length of the fields, whether the fields are numeric, alphanumeric, date, and so forth
- Allowed values for each field, for example, a field representing patient gender may have restrictions that the value of that field can only be "F" or "M"

- Meaning of each field, which is usually a narrative description of what this field represents
- Description of the relationships between entities and whether or not this relationship must always be present
- Description of the application programs that access the database and what operations these applications can perform on the data (i.e., can they change, update, and add data)

The data dictionary, in essence, stores data about data. Without the assistance of the DD, the DBMS would not be able to effectively carry out its functions. For the health information manager, a thorough understanding about the DD is important. One of the potential roles for the health information manager, as is discussed later in this chapter, is the maintenance of the DD.

User Interface

In order to use the various functions of a DBMS, users must be able to communicate easily with the system. Therefore, it is important that a DBMS have a fairly user-friendly interface. Ideally this will be a graphical user interface or icon-based interface.

Transaction Support

In order for data stored in the database to be useful, it must be retrievable to answer queries and support everyday transactions. Transactions, such as registering a clinic patient, admitting an inpatient, formulating a patient bill, or processing a patient's payment, are automated and implemented through application programs. In order for an application program to do its job, it must have access to the data in the database. An important function of a DBMS, therefore, is to provide mechanisms for the application program to manipulate transactions that affect the database.

For example, say a medication needs to be administered to a patient. To complete this transaction several things must take place in the database. First, the medication record for the patient must to be retrieved. Once the modification has occurred in this record, modifications must take place in other files as well. For example, modifications might need to be made in the Pharmacy file for change in patient pharmacy profile; modifications might need to be made in the Utilization Management file because the change might affect the critical-care path of the patient, and so on. All of these steps must be completed when the physician changes the patient's medication order. To execute this transaction, the application program must be able to access the database so that the appropriate records are created and data are transferred to the required files. The facility to do this task is provided through use of a data manipulation language. The DML assists users in directly querying the database, but it is also used by application programmers who embed appropriate DML in their programs to access and manipulate data in the database.

Data Integrity Services

Data integrity means that the same data are consistent and correct throughout all the files in the database. For example, we would expect that the birthdate of a patient would be the same in all the files in which that data element is stored. Integrity is a critical element in any database environment. Without consistent and correct information, the enterprise cannot hope to provide effective services and optimal quality of care.

There are many threats to integrity. First, the integrity of data can be violated when users enter wrong data. For example, a nurse may inaccurately enter the temperature of a patient as 10L instead of 101. In this case, the nurse has mistakenly entered the alpha character "L" for the numeric character "1". The integrity of the data has been violated by a user error. This error could be prevented by implementing certain value constraints in the field.

Another threat to integrity occurs when two or more modifications in the database work well when executed alone, but do not produce the correct results when performed at the same time. A good example is when two admitting clerks are admitting two patients at the same time and assign the two patients to the same bed. A failure in concurrency control has occurred. Before any new transaction can be begun against data in a database, all other transactions against that data must be completed.

A DBMS can help ensure data integrity through the implementation of several constraints. For example, a predefined constraint can be built into the data structure itself. In this instance, the length of data fields might be defined. A patient medical record might be limited to 6 numeric characters with no spaces between the characters. Or the patient's temperature must be recorded using only numeric characters. These constraints are often referred to as *edit checks.*

Other constraints that are used include restricting the range of values that might appear in a field or specifying values that must appear in a field. An example of a constraint on a field value would include limiting the maximum Fahrenheit temperature to 110 or providing a certain range for the dosage of a specific drug. An example of a specific value constraint would be that the patient's gender must be entered as either "F" or "M".

Another type of constraint that can be implemented is based on associations between record fields. For example, a patient's bill cannot be deleted as long as there is an outstanding balance. Another example is that a diagnosis code for hysterectomy cannot be assigned to a male patient.

Concurrent Processing Controls

In enterprise-wide databases there are multiple users accessing the data concurrently. Updating errors can easily occur in this type of environment. Admitting clerks assigning two patients to the same bed is a good illustration of this type of error. Another example may be that the pharmacy department accesses the Master Patient file to retrieve a patient's address. A few seconds before the pharmacy department accessed the patient's record, a clerk in the clinic registration area also accessed the same data and was in the process of updating the address information. In this case, the pharmacy department is reading a record while it is being updated by someone else. The consequence is that the pharmacy department will be looking at invalid data. Essentially, the type of **concurrent processing control** that should be implemented in this case is that when a record update is in progress, no other accesses can be made until the update is completed. This concurrent control is referred to as *locking the record.* Locking an entire record, however, is not efficient. By locking a record, the entire record is not available to other users. For example, say a clerk in the registration area is updating a patient's address. At the same time, the radiology department wants to verify a patient's birthdate and is not interested in the patient's address. Locking the entire patient record would not be efficient because the radiology department would have to wait for access until the registration area completed the record update. A way around this dilemma is to lock fields instead of entire records. In this way, data that are not being updated are still available to other users.

Recovery Services

All systems have the potential of failure or breakdown due to hardware or software problems. A system may malfunction due to a disk crash, a program bug, or other hardware breakdowns. However, in the health-care setting, patient care and other activities must continue regardless of system failure. Therefore, it is imperative that the system can **recover** from such failures and can ensure that data are minimally affected by such shutdowns—the DBMS must recover or reverse the damage done to data and the database during these system crashes.

When a system failure occurs, a transaction may be aborted. For example, if a nurse is entering data on the vital signs of a patient and the transaction is in progress (not completed) when the power supply is unexpectedly interrupted, the DBMS will roll back the transaction and delete any changes made prior to transmission. The DBMS will also alert the nurse once the system is operating again so that the data may be reentered.

If there is a system failure and part of the database itself is lost, a DBMS should have several mechanisms for recovery or returning the database to a correct state. A basic recovery mechanism is to make a backup of the database. The backup copy will be used as a starting point in any recovery activity. Normally, in a health-care facility a backup copy of the database is done on a daily basis.

In addition to making a backup copy of the database, a process called *journaling* is used. Journaling is a procedure whereby all activity against a database is documented in a log or journal. Information in the journal consists of (1) the transaction ID; (2) date and time the transaction took place; (3) type of transaction; (4) record of what data existed before the transaction; and (5) record of what data existed after the transaction. To illustrate how the database journal is used for recovery purposes, let's say that the hospital system shuts down at 7:40 A.M. In addition to a system shutdown, the database has also been destroyed in some way. In order to recover the database, the backup copy would be copied over the version of the database that was operating at the time of the shutdown. Now, because the DBMS has kept a journal of all transactions and has maintained a record of what the data were after the updates, the database can be recreated. This task can be accomplished by updating the backup copy of the database with the updates from the journal that have taken place since the last backup copy was made.

Authorization Controls

It is important that every DBMS provide for data security. In this case, security refers to preventing unauthorized access to the data. There are several mechanisms that can be used to prevent unauthorized (either accidental or intentional) access to the database. Since health information managers are recognized experts in patient confidentiality issues, it is important that they understand the basic mechanisms used to ensure data security.

The most basic method for providing data security is to develop **authorization rules.** The concept on which authorization rules is based is that individuals should only have access to those data that they need to do their job. The level of access and the type of operations that individuals can perform on the data will vary depending on their job position and function. Thus, access to the database and manipulations that can be performed by any given user are usually restricted to the user's subschema or view. In other words, the user is given access to only those data that are designated in the user view.

Authorization rules are frequently implemented through an authorization matrix. The authorization matrix identifies the subject (user), what objects (files, fields, records) the subject can take action on, what actions can be performed by the subject (read, insert, modify, and delete), and what constraints are applied. A sample of an authorization matrix is provided in Figure 6-10.

In this example, authorization is granted to files. However, if authorization was limited to only certain fields, the authorization matrix would indicate this. Authorization for access to and manipulation of data is usually implemented through the use of passwords. Users are assigned a password that must usually be used in conjunction with an individual sign-on code. The password plus the sign-on code then permit access to the database. Further discussion of passwords and related security measures are explored later in this text.

Sometimes the DBMS will not provide the level of security that is desired. In this situation, user-defined procedures must be written by the facility to implement an appropriate security level. It is always better to

User	File	Activity	Constraint
Admitting Clerk	Patient Index	Modify	None
V.P. Finance	General Ledger	Modify	None
Unit Clerk	Patient Index	Read	No Update
	Census File	Modify	None
Emergency Dept. Clerk	Patient Index	Read	No Update

Figure 6-10.   Authorization Matrix

purchase a DBMS that has optimal security measures rather than to absorb the burden of writing appropriate alternate procedures.

When a high level of security is required, the data in the database may be encrypted. **Encryption** means that the data are scrambled by algorithms and make no apparent sense. When a DBMS employs encryption, a legitimate user with appropriate authorization can access the database and the requested data will be decrypted before the user receives it. If an unauthorized user attempts to bypass the DBMS security controls by trying to access the database directly, the interloper will only be able to see encrypted data.

From the above discussion, we can see that several security measures are (or should be) available in a good DBMS. Thus, another advantage of a DBMS over the traditional file processing environment is that basic security measures are readily available for data protection.

Functions of Data and Database Administrators

This chapter has presented a fairly procedural view of the development and implementation of databases and DBMS. Previous sections of the chapter verify that there is a great deal of complexity involved in the development of databases and their management. As we have learned, the data residing in the various enterprise files are an extremely important organizational resource. Without these data and their effective management, the organization could not survive either on an operational or strategic basis. Therefore, it is crucial that the enterprise establish an organizational structure that can manage these data appropriately, which means establishing mechanisms and organizational policy to ensure (1) that databases are appropriately structured to support the organization's strategic thrusts,

(2) that data are consistent and correct, and (3) that data are adequately protected.

When database management systems were first introduced in the 1980s, the tasks relative to data and database management were relegated by default to a variety of people in the organization. The consequence was that there was not very good coordination. As organizations began to recognize the importance of the data resource, formal organizational positions and structures were developed and assigned responsibility for data and database management. These positions encompass the database administration function and are usually headed by the **database administrator** (DBA).

The DBA has traditionally been responsible for both managerial and technical functions of the database administration group. In recent years, however, a distinction is being made between a **data administrator** (DA), who assumes responsibility for the managerial functions, and a database administrator (DBA), who assumes responsibility for the technical functions associated with databases. This dichotomy seems appropriate and, in fact, provides health information managers with an opportunity to assume an important role as a DA in an ever-increasing automated health-care environment. Therefore, in this text, we make a distinction between DA and DBA and emphasize those roles that are most applicable to the health information manager.

Data Administrator Roles

The DA is responsible for the administrative functions associated with data and database management. Among these functions are planning, policy formulation, DBMS evaluation, DD management, and user education. These functions contrast with those normally assumed by the DBA, which are more technical in nature. Among DBA functions are those associated with defining and developing databases, implementing the technical details of a DBMS, planning and monitoring database performance, enforcing security measures, and managing information repositories. The DA position is currently an evolving position in most organizations. As such, the functions of the DA are not clearly defined. In many instances, the DA must be proactive in identifying roles and functions that can be performed to protect the data resource. In today's environment, the DA may report to the director of information systems, or if the organization has a chief information officer (CIO), the DA may report directly to this executive.

Planning Functions

One of the major functions of a DA is to act as an advocate for effective and efficient management of the data resource. In this capacity, the DA may interact with top management (both administrative and clinical) in educating these individuals about the importance of issues such as data integrity and security and how good data planning can support the strategic goals of the organization. The DA should be on the front line in planning information systems that support the overall objectives of the organization. This planning effort is based on developing the conceptual data model for the organization as well as for basic business units of the enterprise. It is the DA's responsibility to ensure that general data and information requirements are identified and transformed into a conceptual data model for the organization. Thus, the DA is responsible for identifying the major entities of an organization, their attributes, and the relationship among entities (see Chapter 5).

Frequently, an enterprise may elect to develop data models using a bottom-up approach, meaning that data models of individual business units will be developed and then combined with other business unit models until eventually a complete enterprise-wide model is developed. The DA should assume major responsibility for this task, including identification of user requirements through interviews, focus groups, and prototype development; and identification of business unit entities, attributes, and relationships. The DA should expect to use CASE (computer-assisted structured engineering) tools to facilitate this process.

A major concern to most enterprises is, "Which information systems should receive development priority?" In other words, given a number of projects that must be done, which ones are the most important? The DA, being familiar with the conceptual and external data models of the organization, may be a participant in helping to determine which application systems should be assigned a high priority. The DA would be expected to work with the DBA in helping to establish an implementation timetable for these systems.

DBMS Evaluation and Selection

The DA may also assume responsibility for the evaluation and selection of a DBMS for an organization. While a team of individuals, both technical and managerial, may participate in DBMS selection and evaluation, the

DA is likely to be responsible for overseeing the process. The evaluation team should consist of user representatives, systems analysts, and software technical specialists. It is the responsibility of the evaluation team to make sure that the DBMS that is selected will support user requirements and the strategic and operational goals of the organization.

Evaluation and selection involves developing a criteria list of features that are desired in a DBMS. The criteria list should include both user-type criteria and technical criteria. Examples of user-type criteria are:

- Does the DBMS have a user-friendly interface?
- Can the DBMS provide quick response to ad hoc queries?
- Does the DBMS provide good security and backup?

Technical criteria examples are:

- What kind of data types are supported by the DBMS—that is, numeric, alpha, date, logical, money, other? Is there support for primary and foreign keys?
- How easy is it to restructure data—for example, add new tables, delete old tables, add columns, delete columns, add new indexes, delete old indexes?
- Are nonprocedural languages such as SQL and QBE supported?
- Are procedural languages such as COBOL and PASCAL supported?
- What type of catalog or data dictionary system is available? Can the DD be integrated with other components of the DBMS?
- What type of concurrency controls does the DBMS have?
- What type of backup and recovery utilities does the DBMS have?
- What type of security implementation is there? Is security implemented through password protection; user subschemas or views; read/write restrictions; encryption?
- What type of support is there for ensuring data integrity?
- What are the structure limitations—that is, how many tables, columns, and rows are supported?
- What is the cost of the system and additional components?
- What is the level of vendor support? What is the cost of vendor support?

- What type of performance can the DBMS provide? Are there comparative tests between this DBMS and others? Will the vendor allow us to run our own tests or benchmarks on the DBMS?
- What documentation is provided with the DBMS? Is this documentation well organized and clearly written? Are on-line tutorials provided?

These items should be weighted or prioritized so that the selection team is clear about what the system should include. After the specifications of a system are identified, the selection team must then evaluate a number of DBMSs against these criteria. Normally this type of evaluation is done by sending a selected number of vendors a formal document called a **request for proposal** (RFP). An RFP is more than a document. It is also an important process.

RFP Document   The RFP is a formal document developed by an organization to assist in making decisions about information systems selection. In this case, it is the selection of a DBMS. The RFP document is distributed to vendors who are expected to provide information to the questions presented in the document about their products. The information gathered through the RFP is essential in helping a DBMS selection and evaluation team make a decision among competing products. It is important that the content of the RFP be complete and accurate because it sometimes also functions as a legal document. Many times the RFP and the response to the RFP by the vendor are included as part of the final contractual arrangement.

The format and content of an RFP document will vary among institutions, but it customarily contains the following sections:

- Cover letter
- Proposal information and format for response
- Conditions of response
- Functional specifications
- Technical requirements
- Implementation requirements
- System costs
- Vendor profile

The RFP customarily begins with a cover letter to prospective vendors requesting them to reply to the proposal that the client has developed. The cover letter or a specific section on proposal information details the intent of the proposal, indicates the timetable for the RFP process, and provides information to the vendor on the format and content of response. Frequently, a disclaimer is also included that ensures the confidentiality of the document—that is, the information in the proposal is considered confidential and no information contained in it can be released without written permission from the organization that developed the RFP.

A section is also included that tells the vendor the format to use in responding to the RFP. For example, in some sections, the RFP may require simple, straightforward, "yes or no" answers. In other sections, the evaluation team may want narrative explanations. The vendor also needs to know whether or not addenda are required (or encouraged) or whether attachments can be included with the response. It is important that the deadline for submission be clearly communicated in this section. The evaluation team must remember that preparing a response to an RFP may take an enormous amount of resources and time on the vendor's part. Therefore, a sufficient amount of time should be allotted for response, usually 4 to 6 weeks.

The RFP includes a profile of the organization. In this section, the background and demographics of the organization are provided. This information helps the vendor to understand the purpose, size, and complexity of the enterprise. Normally information about the mission, goals, organizational structure, and services supported by the organization are provided in the RFP. Additional information about the activity of the organization is also provided. This may include information about the number of admissions/patients seen per day, number of modalities performed, number of employees, number of physicians, and number of departments expected to use the DBMS. This information is helpful to the vendor because it describes the type of activity and volume that a DBMS would be expected to handle. A very important component of this section is a description of the vision that the organization has in regard to data management. This vision is often communicated via a scenario of how the organization expects its DBMS will be used.

Probably the most important section is the functional specification listing the criteria that a DBMS should include. The presentation format is designed so that vendors can indicate whether or not their product currently has the listed function or feature or whether the feature is planned for development. An example of this section appears in Figure 6-11.

Function	Currently Available	Customization Available	Planned Function	Not Available
Front-end user interface				

Data Types Supported
  Alpha
  Numeric
  Date
  Logical
  Money
  Other				

Nonprocedural Languages Supported
  SQL
  QBE
  Other				

Procedural Languages Supported
  COBOL
  C
  PASCAL
  Other				

Data Dictionary Available				

Integrity Services Available
  Field value constraints
  Field length constraints
  Field association constraints				

Concurrency Constraints
  Shared locks
  Exclusive locks
  Deadlock handling				

Figure 6-11. Sample RFP Functional Specifications

The RFP has a technical section with information about the current technical environment, including the hardware, software, and application environment of the organization. In addition, statistics are provided about the activity expected against the database—that is, the number of modifications, deletions, and additions that might be expected per minute or per hour. This information is essential if the vendor (and the client) is to provide accurate projections about DBMS efficiency. The technical section also includes questions to the vendor about the technical environment that must be in place for the DBMS to operate effectively and efficiently. This information is critical to the selection team in determining whether or not current applications can interface with the DBMS easily or whether additional equipment/software will have to be purchased to accommodate the DBMS. It is in this section that vendors are expected to provide performance information about their system and how this performance information was obtained (i.e., what are the benchmarks and testing data used). Samples of system documentation should also be requested including technical and implementation documentation as well as user manuals.

The RFP should address the issues of training and implementation. For example, the vendor should be asked about the kind of training that is provided to users in the organization; how frequent is training; how many individuals can be trained under the standard contract; and so on. A DBMS will be useless if both technical personnel and end-users do not receive appropriate and sufficient training in its operation and use. Questions should also be posed to the vendor about implementation requirements: Who will install the DBMS? Who will be responsible for system testing? Who will be responsible for transfer of existing files to the DBMS? What is the timetable for usual installation? The requesting organization should be clear about "who does what" during the implementation stage. Very often ambiguities concerning vendor versus client responsibilities cause tremendous difficulties during system installation.

Before a client purchases any kind of hardware or software product, a thorough picture of the vendor's stability in the market has to assessed. It would be unfortunate if a client purchased a product from a vendor who subsequently went bankrupt or left the marketplace. This situation would likely leave the client without vendor support or maintenance for the product. Without such support, the client usually must purchase another product. This situation can cause tremendous upheaval within the organizational information infrastructure. Therefore, the client should protect itself as much as possible by doing a thorough background check on the vendor. The RFP should include a request for a vendor profile. In this section, the vendor is asked to supply information about its business organization and financial situation. Information is also requested about the number and demographics of the vendor's installed sites. For example, it would be important to know how many other organizations currently have the product installed, how large these organizations are, and what their performance activity is. Names of the installed sites with a contact person should be provided so that the evaluation team can visit or call these sites. Vendor annual reports should be requested that describe the total revenues for several years and research and development expenditures.

The final sections of the RFP request information about how much the system will cost, what financing arrangements can be negotiated, and contractual material. A system cost schedule should be requested for both lease and purchase options. The cost schedule should list which items are one-time costs, which are annual maintenance costs, and what the projected cost would be over several years—for example, a 5-year period. The schedule may include costs associated with hardware, software, training, custom development, and consulting.

The RFP should also request a copy of all contracts and addenda that are required for the facility to contract to purchase and/or lease the DBMS product. The facility should reserve the right to negotiate the final terms and conditions of the contract. Because the contract binds the facility to certain stipulations, the final contract negotiation should be done with legal consultation.

RFP Process   The RFP is both a document and a process. It is imperative that the RFP process be appropriately managed and monitored. This is where the skills and knowledge of a health information manager prove to be particularly useful. The RFP process technically begins with the analysis of user and system needs and development of functional specifications. Once the technical and functional specifications are developed and are approved by all significant parties within the organization, the RFP document can be prepared. It is important to point out again that the RFP may function as a legal document if it is included as part of the final contract between the client and the vendor. As such, the RFP must be complete and accurate and truly represent the needs of the organization.

The RFP process is like any project. It needs to be managed carefully in order to ensure that all steps take place in a timely manner. The evaluation team must develop a list of steps that need to be accomplished and assign time frames for completion of each. Sample steps in the RFP process might include:

- Identify vendors to which RFP is to be sent.
- Prepare RFP document.
- Distribute RFP document.

- Receive RFP responses.
- Evaluate RFP response/select top vendors.
- Request vendor demonstrations.
- Conduct on-site visits to vendor clients.
- Select the two best vendors.
- Enter contract negotiations.
- Complete contract negotiations.

While the RFP document is being prepared, the selection team must determine who the likely vendors are that can meet the desired specifications. A list of vendors is developed by the team, and it is to these vendors that the RFP is mailed. An ample amount of time (usually 4–6 weeks) is allocated for vendors to respond to the RFP. Once the responses are received, it is the responsibility of the evaluation team to read and evaluate each response against the criteria that were previously developed.

After each proposal is evaluated, a total score for each vendor is calculated. Usually the top two or three vendors are selected to present formal demonstrations of their products. Prior to the demonstrations, the evaluation team should prepare a protocol of questions that they wish to ask the vendor and a protocol of specific features to be demonstrated. After each demonstration, the evaluation team should hold a debriefing to evaluate the demonstration of the product.

It is also valuable for the evaluation team to visit sites where the product is installed. Again, the evaluation team should prepare a protocol of questions and tasks for demonstration at the live site. Formal debriefings should again be held, documenting strengths and weaknesses of the system.

After the demonstrations and site visits are completed, the evaluation team must make a decision on which product to select. All the information gathered through the RFP, demonstrations, and site visits should be considered when making a decision. Once the one or two finalists are selected, legal counsel should be brought in to help conduct contract negotiations.

Data Dictionary Management

A primary function of a DA is responsibility for data dictionary management. A DD is a central storehouse of information about an organization's data. As we saw in the discussion of conceptual, internal, and external model design, the DD is an integral part of a database system where all the data are stored that describe fields, records, files, and file relationships for the organization. An example of the kind of information a DD might store on fields includes:

- Name of each field and any synonyms or aliases it may have. Names for the field that are used in application programs, for example, the formal data dictionary name may be "patient medical record number." However, various departments in the health-care facility may refer to this attribute as "patient number," "medical record number," and so on. One application program may identify this field as "MedRecNo" and another may identify it as "MRNO." All alternative names should be included in the DD.
- Definition of the field, for example, "patient medical record number" definition may be "unique numeric patient identifier that is sequentially assigned at the patient's first registration or admission and that is retained permanently."
- Field type (i.e., alphabetic, numeric, date, etc.).
- Representation (i.e., integer, decimal, etc.).
- Length (number of characters, bytes, decimal positions).
- Value constraints (i.e., what values may be entered in the field).
- Derivation formula if a calculated value.
- Default value, if any.
- Ownership (i.e., users or department responsible for the initial entry of the field value and maintenance of the field value). For "patient medical record number," the users responsible for initial entry of the field value and its maintenance may be the medical record or health information management department.
- Security codes for access and updating.
- Key information (i.e., primary, foreign, or secondary key); relations of the field and rules for updates and deletions.
- Frequency of use and update.
- Location (i.e., if there are multiple databases, in what database is the field located).
- Programs that use the field.
- Screens that use the field.
- Reports that use the field.

The above data describe only fields within a DD. However, a DD must also contain the same type of information about records, files, file relations, user views, programs, reports, screens, and so on. As you can see, the DD is an enormous storehouse of data about data. It is absolutely essential for good management of a database system.

In order for the DD to be useful, information about data must be easy to enter and retrieve. The DD must have facilities to make entry easy and must also have facilities for report generation. There is a wealth of information in the DD that is useful from the standpoint of database management, for example, providing a list of fields in the database; providing a list of aliases for a given field; providing a list of fields by user ownership; cross-reference among field and user views. These types of reports are useful in analyzing various aspects of the database structure, data ownership, security controls, and so on.

Management of an enterprise-wide DD is an enormous task encompassing both entry and update responsibilities as well as analysis functions. Therefore, in a large enterprise, one full-time DA may be assigned with responsibility for this function.

User Training

Another function of the DA may include user training for use of the data dictionary and access to the database. In most instances, routine reports for users are automatically produced by application programs. However, routine reports often do not provide enough information to make decisions. This is particularly true for higher management and executive levels in the organization. Frequently these individuals need data that are not readily available through routine reports. Therefore, various users in the organization or their assistants must know how to access the database to obtain nonroutine information. It is a natural function for the DA to assume responsibility for the training of these users. Depending on the size of the organization, the tasks involving user database training may be a full-time function.

Security

A major concern with any database is its level of security. As an important organizational resource, the database must be protected against intentional or accidental access, modification, or destruction. Think of the critical situation in relationship to patient care that might occur should the database be compromised in any way. It is the DA's responsibility to use the facilities provided by the DBMS to ensure the security of the database.

There are several considerations in regard to database security. First, access to the database must be restricted on a need-to-know basis. This rule applies to both personnel within and outside of the information systems department. The most common way to restrict access is with passwords used in conjunction with identification or sign-on codes. We have already described how access to data can be controlled by the use of user views, subschemas, and profiles and by limiting user access to certain fields, records, or files. In addition, the manipulations that users can perform (access, modify, delete) can also be restricted.

There are issues other than access controls that involve protecting the security of a database. Physical security is also important. For example, access to computer hardware in user areas needs to be constrained. Hospital visitors or other outsiders should not be able to freely access computer terminals or be able to read what is displayed on a terminal screen. Procedures and policies, therefore, regarding physical security are necessary in order to minimize the risk of sabotage and theft.

Other important aspects of security are policies and procedures relating to disaster recovery of the information resource. A disaster can be a system failure caused by hardware or software problems. A disaster can also be a fire, flood, or earthquake. A comprehensive disaster recovery and contingency plan must be developed. Accreditation agencies such as the Joint Commission on Accreditation of Health Care Organizations (JCAHO) require that policies and procedures support a comprehensive plan for disaster recovery. The development and monitoring of such comprehensive plans is the responsibility of the DA or a chief security officer (CSO). Specifics regarding the development of a total security, audit, and control program are discussed in Chapter 9.

Database Administrator Functions

Previously a distinction was made between a DA and a DBA. This distinction may be somewhat arbitrary. However, as organizations become more sophisticated in the management of the information resource, the functions and tasks required to effectively protect this resource are expanding. Therefore, it seems reasonable to separate policy and procedure formulation tasks involving data administration from the more technical tasks of database administration.

The technical tasks that would normally be associated with the DBA include DBMS support, physical database design, analysis of database performance, loading of data into the database for new or converted applications, and testing procedures. These functions would likely be outside the purview of the health information manager and would be assumed by a more technical individual.

Summary

- A database is the collection of data about entities, their attributes, and their relationships among each other.

- The database environment has several advantages over the file processing environment: reduction of data redundancy, better data retrieval, and better data integrity controls.

- A database can use one of several approaches to store and manipulate data. These methods are referred to as the physical data model and include relational, network, hierarchical, and object-oriented approaches.

- The management of database systems is very complex. Management of a database system is accomplished with a software tool called a database management system (DBMS).

- A DBMS provides a number of functions: accessing, updating, and storing data; providing a data dictionary for data descriptions; furnishing a user interface for data manipulation; supporting transaction activities; providing utilities for ensuring data integrity; furnishing concurrent processing controls; providing recovery services; providing security services.

- A data administrator (DA) assumes managerial responsibilities for data and database management. Among these responsibilities are planning functions; DBMS selection and evaluation coordination; data dictionary management; user training development and implementation; data security management.

Review Questions

1. Describe how the conceptual data model for an enterprise supports the development of a physical data model.

2. Explain why an enterprise would want to manage its data through a database environment rather than a file processing environment.

3. Could an enterprise have a database approach to data storage and retrieval without implementing a DBMS? Why or why not?

4. Explain why the functions performed by a data administrator are essential for support of a database environment.

Enrichment Activities

The following activities are provided as enrichment to support the understanding of how database and database management concepts are applied in the work setting.

1. Survey health-care information systems departments in local health-care facilities to determine how many have developed enterprise-wide and/or business-unit conceptual data models. Request copies of the conceptual data models. What do the results of your survey indicate? Are health-care facilities using the data modeling approach for building enterprise-wide databases? Why are they successful in developing conceptual data models? Why aren't they successful?

2. Interview a data administrator or database administrator at a local health-care facility. Obtain a job description for the position. Discuss the responsibilities of the administrator. Are these tasks the same as those described in the text? Are there additional functions that the administrator performs?

3. Obtain a copy of an RFP for selection of a DBMS for a local health-care organization. Analyze the content of the RFP and compare it to the description in this chapter. Are there differences between what is suggested in this chapter and what is contained in your RFP? Why might these differences exist? Do you believe these differences are significant? Would they make a difference in the outcome of the selection process?

4. Arrange to attend a data security committee meeting at a local health-care organization. What are the principal areas of concern in regard to data security at this facility? Are these areas the same as those discussed in this chapter? Has the organization implemented some of the basic security measures discussed in this chapter in regard to database security?

5. Evaluate the functions of a DBMS at a health–care organization in your area. Are these functions adequate? Why or why not? What additional functions, if any, are needed for this facility?

Reference

Codd, E.F. (1970). "A relational model for large shared data banks," *Communications of the ACM 13,(6)*, 377–387.

Chapter 7

Managing Data Quality

Learning Objectives

After completing this chapter, the learner should be able to:

1. Contrast the various definitions of data.
2. Identify the characteristics that constitute data quality.
3. Discuss various methods that can be used to determine the quality of data.
4. Address problems in determining data accuracy. Can accuracy of data ever be determined?
5. Explain practices that can be used to track data quality.
6. Distinguish between the various methods for ensuring data quality.

Key Terms

Data
Data accuracy
Data comprehensiveness
Data consistency
Data currency
Data granularity
Data precision
Data relevancy
Data timeliness

Introduction

The previous chapters present information systems from organizational and architectural views. The evolution of health-care information systems has been studied; the value of information from strategic and operational perspectives has been addressed; and architectures to support more effective and efficient information systems, such as the database environment, have been investigated. This chapter departs somewhat from these more macro issues to examine the nature and quality of the data themselves. No matter how organizationally or architecturally sound an information system might be, the system will be less than optimal if the data that it stores and manipulates are error-ridden. The health-care environment is becoming increasingly more dependent on automated information systems. As reliance on computers has increased, the amount of data that are gathered, stored, and used has escalated at an enormous rate. Today, automated systems and their associated databases are bigger and faster than those of a decade ago. These systems are more functional and complex than their predecessors, allowing end-users to have direct and immediate access to data.

Bigger, faster, and more complex, however, does not necessarily mean better! Remember the old adage associated with computer systems: "If it's garbage in, then it's garbage out." If quality attributes are not inherent in data when they are entered into, and manipulated by, the system, then bigger, faster, and more complex only means more garbage produced faster and distributed to a bigger audience!

Data quality has many more dimensions than "correctness" of data. Data that have inherent quality are data that are comprehensive, current, relevant, accurate, complete, timely, and appropriate. A logical question to ask is, "What is the quality of data in the health-care environment?" The Institute of Medicine (IOM) reported the results of several studies documenting the poor state of various quality dimensions of clinical data in patients' medical records (Dick and Steen, 1991). Tufo and Speidel (1971) evaluated missing data, recording of laboratory results, and incomplete physician narrative. Their results indicated that up to 20 percent of patient charts had data missing. Other studies assessing missing data have revealed similar statistics. Completeness of data, however, is only one aspect of quality. Reliability and consistency are other quality attributes. Other studies cited by the IOM indicate that there are vast disparities in the validity of data. For example, Bentsen (1976) found that 41 percent of patient problems that were identified were not recorded in the patient record. Romm and Putnam (1981) documented that there was up to 80 percent disagreement between the patient record and the verbal content of the physician–patient encounter. Perhaps one of the most outstanding testaments to the unreliability of data was a study conducted by Hsia and colleagues in 1988 that documented an error rate of almost 21 percent in diagnostic coding of patient medical records. Studies done on data quality outside the health-care industry have produced equally dismal results. For example, studies conducted by Johnson, Leitch, and Neter (1981), Laudon (1986), and Morey (1982) reveal error rates between 10 and 75 percent depending on the application.

Thus, there is a significant problem with the quality of data that are gathered, stored, and manipulated. The problem is only magnified as we produce greater amounts of error-ridden data in our bigger, faster, and more complex information systems. A fundamental question is "Can our health-care enterprises withstand the impact of poor-quality data?" Can organizations make good decisions in contracting with managed-care entities when data are incomplete, inconsistent, or unreliable? Can managed-care organizations make appropriate pricing and cost estimates when these decisions are made on data that are incomplete, inconsistent, or unreliable? Can caregivers make appropriate clinical decisions when patient records have incomplete or missing data or when these data are unreliable or unavailable? Can public health officials make projections or track trends in diseases without data that are relevant, comprehensive, accurate, and current? Can we monitor the quality and outcomes of clinical care without data repositories that contain relevant, comprehensive, accurate, complete, reliable, appropriate, and current data?

Historically, health-care enterprises have placed little emphasis on developing processes and assigning responsibility for data quality on an enterprise-wide level. In other words, data quality has fallen through the cracks in most organizations. In today's environment, however, quality data can make a difference in obtaining a strategic or business advantage in the marketplace. It is imperative that health-care enterprises recognize the business advantage of quality data and develop processes, policies, and procedures to protect their value. This is an area of emerging job opportunity for health information managers who can assume roles and functions associated with data quality management.

The Origins of Data Quality

Before we talk about the origins of data quality or identify the dimensions of data quality, we first must understand what **data** are. The literature is replete with definitions of data. For example, data have been defined as unstructured, raw facts, or facts resulting from empirical observations of physical phenomena (Yovits, 1983). This definition, however, is not complete because data are also derived or gathered from sources other than empirical observations of physical phenomena. Blementhal (1969) has defined data as a set of facts. However, for data to be facts, the data must be true or verified. As we know, data entered into and manipulated by information systems are not always true. Another perspective, discussed in Chapter 6, is that data consist of entities, the attributes of these entities, and the relationship among entities. All attributes of entities contain domain fields that constrain the value of entity attributes. Redman (1992) supports this definition of data because it provides a conceptual framework that facilitates evaluation of quality. For example, this definition treats data as a formal, organized, collection that can be studied. It also allows for the evaluation of both the data model (entities and their relationships) and the attributes (values) of the entities. Redman has added an additional parameter in order to assess data quality: the concept of data representation, which is a set of rules for recording data—in other words, the value of a datum will be represented in a certain format and by a specific symbol. Therefore, for our purposes, we will define data as consisting of entities, relationships among entities, and attributes of entities whose values are represented in a specific format and by specific symbols.

Now that a definition of data has been established, we can ask the question, "Where does data quality begin?" Some might say that data quality begins when data are entered into a computer system, for example, when the admitting clerk enters patient demographic data into the hospital information system; or when the nurse enters a patient's vital signs into the nursing information system; or when the radiology technician enters treatment data into the radiology information system. Others might say that data quality begins when data entered into a computer system are "checked" or "edited" for appropriate field values. We studied some of these procedures in Chapter 6 in our discussion of field edit checks and data dictionary maintenance. Others might say that data quality begins with policies and procedures that oversee the maintenance of corporate databases, for example, procedures to limit access and the modification made on data, consistency checks, and so on. Others might say that quality begins with the development of the conceptual data model.

What precedes data entry? What precedes database design? What precedes development of policies and procedures for database management? What precedes all of these steps is the actual work process that creates and uses data. In other words, data quality begins with data creation—the underlying processes that create and use data. Therefore, any program that attempts to ensure data quality must include the study of the work processes that create and use data.

The data modeling approach described in Chapter 5 provides a methodology for studying such work processes. By identifying the entities, attributes, attribute values, and relationships among entities for a given work process, the basic task of defining data has been accomplished. In other words, because we have studied the work processes of the user, we can be relatively assured that the data we are collecting and storing will meet user needs—that is, the data are relevant, sufficiently comprehensive, complete, and appropriate. Once the data modeling task has been completed, other activities can be implemented to help ensure that the data contain other necessary dimensions of quality such as accuracy, currency, and reliability.

Characteristics of Data Quality

The characteristics of data quality are frequently described in terms of data relevancy, completeness, accuracy, precision, accessibility, and timeliness. Many times the term *integrity* is used to refer to the entire set of characteristics associated with data quality. Probably one of the more complete views of the dimensions of data quality is presented by Redman (1992). His model is based on assessing the characteristics of the end-users' view (i.e., subschema). In other words, quality is integrated into the process of developing the end-users' subschema or conceptual view of the data. If the subschema adequately portrays the process, then quality is automatically derived. An adaptation of these characteristics is presented below.

First, a prerequisite to data quality is **data relevancy,** which means the data are meaningful to the performance of the process or application for which they are collected. For example, let's take the view or subschema of a clinic admitting clerk. One of the processes that an admitting clerk performs is the collection of patient demographic information so that the patient can be uniquely identified during current and subsequent admissions. We would say that the collection of data items such as patient name, date of birth, and sex are relevant for the process of being able to uniquely identify a patient. On the other hand, collection of data items such as the patient's hobbies or names of the patient's pets would be totally irrelevant or nonessential. Therefore, when the user subschema is developed, it is necessary to identify all relevant data and exclude data that are not essential.

A second characteristic of data quality is that data items should be easily obtainable or legal to collect. For example, a health-care provider may need to collect data about a patient's race or age in order to make an adequate diagnosis. However, the collection of such information by an employee in the human resources management department may be illegal. Another example would be the collection of data for tracking patients. Let's say the radiology department is interested in collecting data to determine where backlogs are occurring in the department. This will mean collecting data on the time the patient arrived in the department; the time the patient entered the x-ray exam room; the time the x-ray was taken; the time the patient left the x-ray room; the time the x-ray was interpreted; the time the patient was discharged from the x-ray department. The collection of these data could be time-consuming and interfere with the usual work tasks of the radiology employees. Because of the extensive documentation process that does not fit into the regular work flow of the department employees, it is likely that the data collected would be incorrect. In this instance, the data are not easily obtainable. It would probably be better to have the management engineering department track patients for a limited amount of time, rather than to collect these data on a permanent basis.

As discussed in Chapters 5 and 6, the definition of each entity and attribute must make sense in the context of the process or application to be performed. It is important that clear definitions be provided so that current and future data users will know what the data mean. A good example is the use of diagnostic codes in patient abstracting systems. Let's say that a physician wants to do a study of all acute myocardial infarction patients treated in the past 25 years. If the data analyst searched the diagnostic index back 25 years using today's ICD-9 code, the data that would be retrieved would likely be incorrect, because several different coding systems have been used during this time period and the code for acute myocardial infarction would be different in each classification. If the health-care facility has not kept track of the coding classifications used and their period of use, the task of collecting the correct data will be difficult.

Another prerequisite to data quality is that all data items that are required should be included. This is usually referred to as **data comprehensiveness** and has to do with the scope of the data collected. Usually, we will want to build as much flexibility as possible into our subschema views, anticipating future data needs. This is particularly true if there is a high probability that some external factor will influence our data requirements. A good example is today's pressure for outcome data. Organizations that foresaw the trends developing in the health-care environment and began collecting these types of data several years ago are at a distinct advantage over their competitors today.

Data granularity should be **appropriate**—that is, the attributes and their values should be defined at the correct level of detail. Patient name is a good example of the need for detail. Let's say that we want to retrieve data on a patient named Mr. Jones. If we enter only the name "Jones," we will probably get several, if not hundreds, of listings for "Mr. Jones." In order to better retrieve data for our specific Mr. Jones, we need to define his name at a greater level of detail. For example, we will want to use his first name and most likely his middle initial in order to easily retrieve the data we need. Another example of data granularity is a patient's temperature reading. In order for the data to be useful, we would want to define the level of detail to the first decimal point (i.e., 101.1, 101.2, 101.3, etc.). From a clinical perspective there is a significant difference between a temperature of 101.1 and 101.9, so it is important that we collect data to the first decimal point to provide appropriate data granularity .

In Chapter 6, mention was made that acceptable values or value ranges should be defined for each attribute. These values should be just large enough to support the application or process. This concept is referred to as **data precision**. For example, we would want to limit the range of values of the gauge of a needle that was used or inserted into a catheter. The range of value or precision in this case might be 16 to 22. Another example is the unit dosage of insulin that can be ordered for a patient. The value range or precision in this case might be 1 to 12. As you can see, making the data as precise as possible helps to reduce data error, particularly if these values are enforced through automatic edit checks.

Data timeliness is also an important quality concern. The need for timely data, however, is context dependent. For example, in the critical-care unit of a hospital, data required for patient care need to be current or timely. In fact, the timeliness of data is so important in this context that they may need to be collected and reported on a second-by-second basis. On the other hand, data used for the routine examination of a patient during a yearly physical will not have to be as timely as that in the critical-care unit. From a management decision-making perspective, another example of the context-dependent nature of data timeliness is that data for operational decisions need to be more current than data for strategic decision making. Thus, the need for data timeliness will depend on the individual situation and user subschema.

Data currency is an important attribute of data quality, referring to whether a datum is up to date. As the ICD-9 coding example demonstrates, data values change over time. What a certain datum value meant 10 years ago may not be the same today. A datum value is up to date if it is current for a specific point in time. It is outdated if it is incorrect at a certain point of time but was correct at some preceding time.

Data consistency is another attribute of data quality. We would expect that if attributes overlap entities (i.e., the same attribute is in more than one entity), the value of those attributes would be the same or consistent. For example, in the emergency department example in Chapters 5 and 6, several entities had overlapping attributes—that is, patient number. We would expect that the value of patient number would be the same across these entities. A good example of inconsistency is the file processing environment scenario in Chapter 6. Recall that many of the attribute values shared by several files in that example were different from each other or inconsistent.

Another type of inconsistency occurs when two related (but not identical) data items do not agree. For instance, a hysterectomy is related to the sex of a patient. A female patient has a hysterectomy. An inconsistency would arise between these related data if it were documented that a male patient had a hysterectomy.

Data should be accurate. If a patient's sex is male, then this should be accurately recorded in the patient's record. If the patient's name is Russell James, then this should be correctly documented. Saying that data ought to be accurate and determining the level of accuracy are two different things. In order to determine **data accuracy,** we must know the correct value. For example, say that a white blood count was reported as 10,000 for a certain patient who is suspected of having an infection. How do we know whether or not this datum value is accurate for this patient? Unless there is some other source for verifying the accuracy of this reported laboratory result, we have no direct way of measuring its accuracy. We can only hope to increase the accuracy of data through database management techniques such as the use of field value constraints and consistency checks.

An attribute that affects data quality, but that is not inherent in the data themselves, is the format by which data are presented to the end-user. Format in this instance does not refer to screen layouts or printed reports. Rather, it refers to the symbols used to convey the meaning of the data. For instance, formats may include use of character strings, icons, images, graphics, metaphors, or color. Laboratory test results are usually represented by character strings. However, lab test results may be highlighted by color when they are not within normal limits. We are all familiar with the use of icons. Virtually every microcomputer application today communicates with end-users through the use of icons. Icons are special symbols or "pictures" that represent categories of data or commands or features of an application program. Examples of icons used in medical documentation are the male ($\male$) and female ($\female$) symbols. Metaphors are becoming increasingly more popular in representing the value of data. A metaphor in this case is the use of a graphic as an implied comparison to some datum or item. For example, to represent the value of a patient's temperature, a graphic of an oral thermometer whose mercury reading is positioned at the patient's temperature reading might be used as a graphical metaphor. No matter what data representation is used, it is important that the method be appropriate to the user's needs and can be easily interpreted. Flashiness should never replace useful data representation.

Determining the Quality of Data

Now that we know what constitutes data quality, how do we go about ensuring that these attributes exist in our organizational data? A five-level approach incorporated into a total data quality management plan can be implemented to manage data quality in organizations: (1) determining data quality requirements; (2) developing, measuring, and tracking systems to monitor data quality; (3) analyzing the results of data monitors; (4) improving processes that create and use data; and (5) implementing information system data control features. This approach is represented in Figure 7-1.

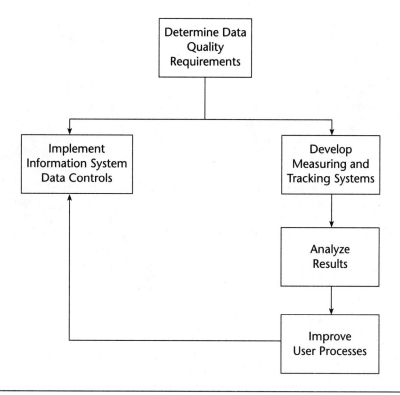

Figure 7-1.   Model for Data Quality Assurance

Determining Data Quality Requirements

The first step in development of an overall data quality program is to know what the requirements for data quality are. For example, does the patient ID number in the organizational database need to be correct 100 percent of the time? How timely must data be for executive-level decision making—that is, can the data be 1 day old, 1 week old, or 1 month old? How complete must the data on population demographics be in order to determine trends for managed-care contract decision purposes? These data quality questions should be addressed at the time the user subschema of the data model is developed—that is, at the point where data quality begins.

The essential process for identifying data quality requirements consists of the following steps: (1) identify the user requirements; (2) identify the data quality attributes and the level of these for each requirement; and

(3) translate quality requirements into technical performance requirements. The emergency room example used previously will provide the scenario for examining how this process is carried out.

A patient arrives at the emergency department on a walk-in basis. The ED registration clerk registers the patient. Through the registration process, the clerk gathers the following data: patient name; address; birthdate; sex; insurance carrier name; insurance carrier number and group number; insurance carrier address; chief complaint; family physician; mode of arrival; time of arrival; and social security number. After registration, the patient is seen by the triage nurse. The nurse notes the time that the patient is seen, confirms the patient's chief complaint, gathers additional information about the patient's condition, history, and vital signs, and assigns the patient a priority level. The patient is then put in a queue according to priority level and is seen by the ED physician.

When the user's subschema model is being developed, users should not only be queried about the process that takes place, but should also be asked about the quality requirements of the data and what these data are used for. For example, the registration clerk may say that it is absolutely essential that the patient's name and birthdate be correct 100 percent of the time. Perhaps the ED administrative director says that she needs to be able to retrieve data on an ad hoc basis to study the department patient flow and productivity. Thus, the ED director may say that it is essential that the time of arrival and the time first seen by the triage nurse be documented. However, the "exactness" of these times probably does not have to be perfect, perhaps being within a minute or two of the actual time. The triage nurse may say that the patient's demographic data need only be complete 80 percent of the time. Table 7-1 is a matrix that shows how each user views the quality attributes of the data.

User and the data items are listed in table columns. Quality attributes are listed in table rows. Note that these attributes may change from context to context. For example, in some contexts we would want to include the attribute of currency and perhaps in others this attribute would not be included. The quality attributes that are included will depend on the user context. Notice that each user has rated each quality attribute as high, medium, or low. The matrix shows how the registration clerk, nurse, and ED director differ on their opinions about the level of the data quality attributes.

Table 7-1. Quality Attributes by Data

Quality Attributes	Clerk		Nurse		Director	
	Pt. Demographic Data Collected at Registration	Chief Complaint Collected at Registration	Pt. Demographic Data Collected at Registration	Chief Complaint Collected at Registration	Pt. Demographic Data Collected at Registration	Chief Complaint Collected at Registration
Accuracy	H	L	H	H	H	H
Completeness	H	L	L	H	H	H
Consistency	H	L	H	H	H	H
Currency	H	L	L	H	H	H
Timeliness	H	L	M	H	H	H

H = high; M = medium; L = low.

After the data quality attributes have been matched with the user requirements, the next step is to translate these into technical requirements. Certainly differences in user opinions about the importance of each quality attribute will need to be reconciled. Table 7-2 presents a matrix of the translation of the user requirements into technical requirements.

Once the data quality attributes have been identified and translated into technical performance requirements, various information system controls can be implemented to help ensure compliance. For instance, in the example above, if demographic information had to be complete 100 percent of the time, then an automatic system constraint could be implemented that would require all fields to be completed before the data entry clerk could go on to another screen and/or close the record.

Measuring and Tracking Data Quality

Once data quality requirements have been identified, a system for measuring and tracking whether or not these requirements are being met must be designed. Since we know that data quality begins with the user process, one approach to tracking and monitoring is to begin an examination of records at the process level. A table of the various fields and processes they affect can be constructed. Let's use a simplistic model of a patient being

Table 7-2.   User Requirements with Technical Specification

User Requirements	Technical Specification
Collect patient demographic data at registration	The collection of demographic data occurs at the time the patient presents to the emergency department. The content consists of patient name; address; birthdate; sex; insurance carrier name; insurance carrier number and group number; insurance carrier address; chief complaint; family physician; mode of arrival; time of arrival; and social security number.
	Patient name, birthdate, and sex must be complete 100 percent of the time. Other fields should be complete 98 percent of the time. All fields should be accurate 100 percent of the time.
Document chief complaint at time of registration	The documentation of chief complain occurs at the time of registration and is verified by the triage nurse.
	Chief complaint must be complete 100 percent of the time; it must be accurate 100 percent of the time.

Table 7-3.   Data Fields by End-User Process

	Registration Process	**Nursing Assessment Process**	**Lab Order-Entry Process**	**Pharmacy Order-Entry Process**	**Patient File**	**Encounter File**
Patient Number	Created	x	x	x	x	x
Patient Lname	Created	x	x	x	x	x
Patient Fname	Created	x	x	x	x	x
Patient Minitial	Created	x	x	x	x	x
Birth Date	Created	x	x	x	x	x
Patient Sex	Created	x	x	x	x	x

admitted to an acute-care facility for our example. Table 7-3 shows the fields that each of the end-user processes have in common. In other words, each of these processes uses several of these fields. This table gives us a view of where data are created and where they can be subsequently modified, allowing us to track individual records through various processes to see how the data might change. The table also shows in what database files the data are stored. This information will help us later when we look at the consistency of data among the various data files and/or databases.

Once such a matrix has been developed , actual records can be tracked. This is usually accomplished through selecting and electronically tagging a random sample of records. A printout of data on the activity of each record as it crosses the various processes is created. Table 7-4 shows such a printout of the activity for one record across all the four processes.

Table 7-4.   Record Activity across Processes

	Registration Process	**Nursing Assessment Process**	**Lab Order-Entry Process**	**Pharmacy Order-Entry Process**	**Patient File**	**Encounter File**
Patient Number	456789	457890	457890	457890	457890	457890
Patient Lname	Hunt	Hunt	Hunt	Hunt	Hunt	Hunt
Patient Fname	Robert	Robert	Robert	Robert	Robertt	Robert
Patient Minitial	J	J	J	J	J	J
Birth Date	03-21-48	032148	03-21-48	03-21-48	032148	032148
Patient Sex	Male	Male	Male	Male	Male	Male

Notice that the patient number is different in the registration process than in the other processes. This difference in value indicates an inconsistency in data for some reason. Since we would not normally expect this field to be changed, we would want to investigate why this difference exists—in other words, what went wrong at the process level to create this inconsistency. Note also that the birthdate field has differences in format presentation. Since the actual values of the birthdate are not different, we would not be concerned with the presentation format differences.

Analyzing Results of Monitoring and Tracking

Once monitoring and tracking systems have been put in place, the results of these systems need to be analyzed. The analysis should attempt to determine if the results indicate trends or if aberrant behavior exists. Taking the example above, the data over many records might indicate that the patient number is frequently changed during the nursing assessment. This would be a trend. Let's say, however, that the patient number was changed in only one record and that occurrence happened during the nursing admission process. This would be called an aberrant behavior. Trends in data more likely show that there is a problem with an underlying process. An aberrant data point more likely means that something outside the process intervened to cause the problem. Distinguishing between trends and specific instances of deviation is important from the standpoint of analyzing the underlying cause of the problem. To help assess whether results from monitoring and tracking systems are trends or not, statistical quality control measures used in quality improvement can be applied. Thus, it is important to uncover the underlying causes of poor data quality and then to correct these causes.

Improving Processes That Use and Create Data

After results of monitoring and tracking have been analyzed, action must be taken to remediate or correct the causes contributing to poor data quality. If the change of the patient number in the above example was determined to be a trend, occurring frequently across many records, then we would want to look at the process of nursing assessment. What in this process is causing the patient number to be changed? The cause could be a human error where a nursing assistant is changing or editing a field that should not be changed. It could also be an information systems error. Perhaps the interface between the registration system and nursing system is malfunctioning in some manner. To determine the cause of such errors, the entire process must be reviewed. Once causes have been identified, it is necessary to implement changes that will improve the process associated with data creation or use.

Implementing Information Systems Data Control Features

In Chapter 6, the characteristics of a DBMS and the functions of a data administrator were discussed. Many of the functions of a DBMS are geared toward providing data quality. One of the first defenses against poor data quality is the maintenance of a data dictionary. As we learned, a DD is a central storehouse of information about an organization's data. The DD stores data that describe fields, records, files, and file relationships. Such a storehouse is necessary from the standpoint of cataloging what data exist and how they are used. Since there are probably thousands of data fields for any given organization, thousands of processes, and thousands of files, without the assistance of a data dictionary it would be impossible to put together the type of matrix found in Table 7-4. Thus, the data dictionary is a basic element in assisting with data quality.

The DBMS can also impose various constraints and edits to help ensure data quality. As we saw previously, value ranges can be incorporated into the data dictionary for data fields. This places a constraint on the value of the data that can be placed in the system. Logical consistency checks or field association checks can also be incorporated to ensure data accuracy. Remember the hysterectomy example. A logical consistency check would recognize that there was a relationship between the sex of a patient and a hysterectomy procedure. This check would not allow a hysterectomy to be documented in a male patient's record.

While various DBMS functions can be used to promote data quality, these functions in and of themselves are not sufficient to ensure data integrity. Therefore, a combination of methods must be implemented and managed by the data administrator.

Summary

- Historically, health-care enterprises have placed little emphasis on developing processes and assigning responsibility for data quality on an enterprise-wide level. In today's environment, however, quality data can make a difference in obtaining a strategic or business advantage in the marketplace. Therefore, it is imperative that health-care enterprises recognize the business advantage of quality data and develop processes, policies, and procedures to protect their value.

- There are several definitions of data. Some of these emphasize that data are a set of facts resulting from empirical observations of physical phenomena. Another view of data is that they consist of entities, relationships among entities, and attributes of entities whose values are represented in a specific format and by specific symbols.

- Data quality begins at the origin of the creation and usage of data. Therefore, any program that attempts to ensure data quality must include the study of the work processes that create and use data.

- Data quality has several characteristics: relevancy, accessibility, timeliness, currency, consistency, accuracy, precision, and completeness.

- A multistep approach can be used to determine and help ensure data quality: determining data quality requirements; developing measuring and tracking systems to monitor data quality; analyzing results of the data monitors; improving processes that use and create data; and implementing information system data control features.

Review Questions

1. Discuss the various definitions of data. What are the strengths and weaknesses of each definition?

2. The chapter states that the quality of data begins with the processes that create and use data. Explain the meaning of this statement. Give examples of where this view holds true. Can you think of any examples where this view would not hold true?

3. Describe the characteristics of data quality. Are all of these characteristics essential in every situation? Explain why or why not.

4. Explain how you would go about determining the quality of data in a health-care facility. What are the strengths and weaknesses of the method you are proposing?

5. What type of system would you implement in a health-care facility to protect the quality of data? How effective and efficient would this system be?

Enrichment Activities

1. Take five patient medical records. Develop a matrix of quality attributes and data items for these records. Review the records and tabulate the results about the quality of data in these records. What does your analysis show? Can data quality be effectively measured using this process? Why or why not?

2. Obtain five or six different printouts of data from a health-care facility. Develop a matrix of quality attributes for data items that are duplicated across the reports. Review these data items against the quality attributes you have selected. What do your results indicate? Were you able to adequately determine data quality in this instance? Why or why not? What additional information would you need to make determinations about data quality in this instance?

References

Bentsen, B.G. (1976). The accuracy of recording patient problems in family practice. *Journal of Medical Education, 51,* 311.

Blumenthal, S.C. (1969). *Management information systems.* Englewood Cliffs, NJ: Prentice-Hall.

Dick, Richard S., and Steen, Elaine B. (eds.) (1991). *The Computer-based patient record: An essential technology for health care.* Washington, DC: National Academy Press.

Hsia, D.C., Drushat, W.M., Fagan, A.B., Tebbutt, J.A., and Kusserow, R.P. (1988). Accuracy of diagnostic coding for Medicare patients under the prospective-payment systems. *New England Journal of Medicine, 318,* 352–355.

Johnson, R., Leitch, R.A., and Neter, J. (1991, April). Characteristics of errors in accounts receivables and inventory audits. *Accounting Review, 56* (2), 270–293.

Laudon, K.C. (1986, January). Data quality and due process in large interorganizational record system. *Communications of the ACM, 29* (1), 4–18.

Morey, R.C. (1982, May). Estimating and improving the quality of information in a MIS. *Communications of the ACM, 25* (5), 337–342.

Redman, T.C. (1992). *Data quality management and technology.* New York: Bantam Books.

Romm, F.J., and Putnam, S. M. (1981). The validity of the medical record. *Medical Care, 6,* 618–630.

Tufo, H.M., and Speidel, J.J. (1971). Problems with medical records. *Medical Care, 9,* 509–517.

Yovits, M.C. (1983). Information and data. In *Encyclopedia of computer science and engineering,* 2nd ed. New York: Van Nostrand Reinhold, pp. 715–717.

Chapter 8

Data Retrieval and Analysis

Learning Objectives

After completing this chapter, the learner should be able to:

1. Explain the use of data manipulation languages such as SQL and QBE.

2. Distinguish between the purposes of data definition, data manipulation, and data control commands in a data manipulation language.

3. Discuss what steps must be taken to organize a meaningful data analysis project. Why are each of these steps important?

4. Distinguish between nominal, ordinal, and interval data, providing examples of each.

5. Distinguish between discrete and continuous interval data.

6. Discuss descriptive measures that are used to describe data.

7. Explain the purpose of a measure of association and dispersion. Discuss the various measures that can be used to analyze data.

8. Discuss what is meant by statistical significance. Identify various statistical techniques that are used to determine statistical significance and differences among group means.

9. Discuss the more common graphical techniques that are used for data presentation.

10. Provide examples of ways that graphical presentations can be distorted.

Key Terms

Bar Chart

Continuous Data

Discrete Data

Frequency Distribution

Histograms

Interval Data

Line Graphs

Mean

Measures of Central Tendency

Measures of Dispersion

Median

Mode

Nominal Data

Ordinal Data

Polygons

Query by Example

Standard Deviation

Statistical Significance

Structured Query Language

Variance

Introduction

Data retrieval and analysis are two of the important domains of practice of the health information manager (HIM). While these domains have historically been important functions for the HIM, they are becoming increasingly more significant in today's environment. The current health-care climate requires that decision makers have access to data about the competitive environment and their organization in order to assess both threats and opportunities. In addition, the consumer of health-care services is demanding more and more information about the appropriateness and quality of care. In the ever-growing managed-care environment, the availability of quality data is essential for making sound decisions and projections about patient profiles, required resources, utilization, and quality of care.

Paradoxically, while there is a great need for the retrieval and analysis of data, there are also significant barriers to data access and a lack of sophisticated knowledge about the techniques for data analysis and presentation. Thus, this is an opportunity for the HIM to transform and update previous skills and knowledge to fit the needs of the current environment. This chapter provides an introduction to three major areas concerned with data retrieval and analysis. The first section deals with tools for extracting data from relational databases. SQL and QBE, which are mentioned briefly in Chapter 5, are discussed in more depth in this chapter. The second section deals with an introduction to basic statistics and the use of statistical software packages for data analysis. The final section introduces concepts associated with data presentation techniques.

Retrieval and Manipulation of Data

The primary way data are retrieved and manipulated in a database is through the use of a data manipulation language (DML). There are several data manipulation languages. As we learned previously, a DML assists in performing several types of tasks associated with a database management system (DBMS). A principal task is querying the database—in other words, extracting or retrieving data from the database. Two of the more popular data manipulation languages are **structured query language** (SQL) and **query by example** (QBE).

Structured Query Language

SQL was developed by IBM in the 1970s under the name SEQUEL. The name was changed to SQL in 1980 and was approved as an ANSI (American National Standards Institute) standard in 1986. SQL is used as a DML for relational DBMS. Often, it is associated with mainframe DBMS, including IBM's popular DB2 product. The SQL standard was updated in 1989 and a new version, SQL2, is currently in review.

In SQL there are three categories of commands: those for data definition, data manipulation, and data control. Using data definition commands, SQL allows the user to create tables (files), delete tables, and create views from the database. The data manipulation commands allow the end-user to retrieve data, add new rows (records), change existing rows, and delete rows from a table. The control commands provide a mechanism to control access to the data as well as aborting incomplete transactions. The categories of commands—data definition, data manipulation, and data control—should be somewhat familiar to the learner. Recall that these concepts were presented in Chapter 6 in the discussion about the functions that a DBMS should perform. These included functions associated with creating the database, manipulating the data, and providing integrity controls. In this section, we describe in more detail how these functions are carried out through a specific data manipulation language called SQL. Table 8-1 provides a summary of the functions that can be performed by SQL along with associated commands.

To provide a preview of how SQL is used, we will use the emergency department example from previous chapters. Figure 8-1 shows all the tables for the ED database.

Data Definition: Creating the Database

Before any data can be put in a database, the tables (files) in the database must be created. To create a database table using SQL, the command CREATE TABLE is used along with the table name. After creating the table, we

Table 8-1. SQL Commands

Functions	AVG, COUNT, MAX, MIN, SUM
Operations	CLOSE, COMMIT, DECLARE, FETCH, INSERT, OPEN, ROLLBACK, SELECT, UPDATE
Predicates	LIKE, NULL ORDER BY, UNION
Schema Definition Language	CREATE SCHEMA, CREATE VIEW, TABLE
Basic Referential Integrity	CHECK, FOREIGN KEY, UNIQUE
Security	GRANT, REVOKE

Payer Table

Payer ID

Residence Table

Street	**City**	**State**	**Zip**	**MR#**

Patient Table

MR#	**Lname**	**Fname**	**Middle Initial**	**Sex**	**Birthdate**

Encounter Table

En. #	**Date**	**Arrival Time**	**Mode of Arrival**	**Chief Complaint**	**Disposition**	**Discharge Date**	**Discharge Time**	**Dx Code**	**MR#**

Employee Table

Employee ID	**En #**

Physician Table

Physician ID	**En #**

Test/Treatment Table

Test #	**Time Ordered**	**Time Completed**	**En #**

Figure 8-1. Relational Database Tables: Emergency Department Database

must define to the database the attributes (fields) within the table and identify the characteristics of each attribute. The following example shows how the patient table would be created and defined using SQL.

```
CREATE TABLE PATIENT
    MR#            INTEGER (7),
    LNAME          CHAR (20),
    FNAME          CHAR (15),
    MINITIAL       CHAR (1) ,
    SEX            CHAR (1),
    BIRTHDATE      DATE
```

Note that in the above example the physical characteristics for each column in the table have been defined. For example, MR# is 7 integers (numbers) long, LNAME is 20 characters long, and so on. A special characteristic DATE indicates that a date format will be entered for this attribute.

After our table has been created, we can now populate it by putting data into the table. Figure 8-2 displays a populated patient table.

Populated Patient Table

MR#	Lname	Fname	Middle Initial	Sex	Birthdate
6789076	Michaels	Frances	J	F	04-21-56
7654345	Sevelle	Constance	M	F	01-03-51
8900234	Ludwig	Joan	M	F	10-14-58
7623451	Sandness	Johnathan	F	M	06-05-55
8745231	McBain	Sean	D	M	03-17-46
8765098	Brodnick	Melanie	S	F	02-09-64
6543219	Osborn	Carol	A	F	08-23-64
7645231	McGee	Travis	J	M	05-06-74
7634521	Moon	Allen	K	M	03-14-60
7834561	Rugh	James	W	M	07-21-56

Figure 8-2.   Populated Patient Table

Data Manipulation: Querying the Database

Since we now have a populated table, we can make some queries against the table using SQL. Let's say that we want to make a simple query asking the DBMS to retrieve the last name of all the patients in the table. The following command would execute this query:

> SELECT MR#, LNAME
>   FROM PATIENT

The response to the above query would be a listing of all the patients and their respective medical record numbers. Notice that the SQL command SELECT was used followed by the attributes of interest. Note also that the query includes the name of the table "Patient" to tell the DBMS where (in what table) these data are located.

What if we wanted a list of only the patients who were males? SQL would handle this query using the following command:

> SELECT MR#, LNAME
>   FROM PATIENT
>   WHERE SEX = M.

Notice that we have again used the command SELECT to direct the DBMS to retrieve the list of attributes MR# and LNAME. However, this time the command specifies that only male patients are of interest. This constraint on the query is done by using the command WHERE with the arithmetic operator "=" and then the value of male, which in this case is "M". The response to the above query would provide the following list:

7623451	Sandness
8745231	McBain
7645231	McGee
7634521	Moon
7834561	Rugh

Let's say that we wanted to refine the above list and have it put in alphabetical order. The following command would be used:

```
SELECT MR#, LNAME
    FROM PATIENT
    WHERE SEX = M
    ORDER BY LNAME
```

Notice that the above command is exactly like the previous one, except in this case we have asked the DBMS to order or sort the names alphabetically. This is accomplished by the command ORDER followed by the attribute on which we wish to sort. The result to this query would look like the following:

8745231	McBain
7645231	McGee
7634521	Moon
7834561	Rugh
7623451	Sandness

Often in queries comparison operators are used. Comparison operators include the following symbols: =, <, >, <=, >=, <>. One of the above queries used the comparison operator = when we were requesting a list of male patients. Another example of the use of comparison operators is the following query: "Print a listing of all patients with a medical record number equal to or greater than 8000000. In SQL this query would be represented by the following command:

```
SELECT MR#, LNAME
    FROM PATIENT
    WHERE MR# >= 8000000
```

The response to this query would provide the following list:

8745231	McBain
8765098	Brodnick
8900234	Ludwig

In SQL, multiple comparison operators can be used in the same query. This is accomplished by connecting two or more simple conditions together using the words AND, OR, and NOT. This type of query is referred to as a compound condition. For example, let's say that we wanted a listing of all male patients who had a medical record number equal to or greater than 8000000. The query would be formulated in the following way:

```
SELECT MR#, LNAME
    FROM PATIENT
    WHERE MR# ≥ 8000000
    AND SEX = M
```

The response to this query would provide the following patient:

    8745231   McBain

SQL also has several built-in functions. These commands are included in Table 8-1 in the first row. These built-in functions perform calculations such as counting, averaging, adding, and identifying minimum and maximum values. For instance, say that we were interested in knowing how many female patients we had in our database. The SQL query would be formulated like the following:

```
SELECT COUNT(SEX)
    FROM PATIENT
    WHERE SEX = F
```

This query is similar to those that we have already seen. The SELECT command is used with the COUNT command. In this query we have specified that the attribute we wanted counted is SEX. The query is continued like the other queries, indicating that the DBMS must look in the PATIENT table. To be sure that only female patients are counted, we have use the conditional operator "=" with the attribute SEX. The response to this query would be a number count of 5 female patients.

So far we have only been working with one table. What if the data we need are in two or more tables? How does SQL handle this kind of query? We will need to populate another table from the emergency department example. Figure 8-3 is an example of the populated residence table. To demonstrate extracting data from two tables, let's say that we want a listing of patient names who come from a specific geographical area, in this case zipcode 34567. To perform this query in SQL we would issue the following command:

Street	City	State	Zip	MR#
456 Pine St	Anytown	OH	34567	6789076
78923 Arlington	Anytown	OH	34789	7654345
18381 Green Castle	Anytown	OH	34567	8900234
3254 Highland Dr	Anytown	OH	34567	7623451
24612 Maple Valley Rd	Anytown	OH	34221	8745231
3801 Alaska	Anytown	WA	99880	8765098
5721 Blake Place	Anytown	CA	92334	6543219
3201 Bluff Way	Anytown	OH	34228	7645231
6792 8th Ave	Anytown	OH	34227	7634521
18381 Hillcrest	Anytown	OH	34789	7834561

Figure 8-3.   Populated Residence Table

```
SELECT LNAME, ZIP
   FROM PATIENT, RESIDENCE
   WHERE ZIP = 34567
```

As we can see, the standard format is used. The SELECT command is followed by the two attributes of interest, in this case last name and zip. After identifying what specific data we are interested in, the next command indicates in what tables these data are located. In this case, data are from the tables PATIENT and RESIDENCE. Note also that we have used a comparison operator to narrow our search to only those patients in zip-code 34567. The result of our query would be:

```
Michaels     34567
Ludwig       34567
Sandness     34567
```

The previous examples demonstrate how SQL is used to extract data from the database. There are many more adaptations and uses of commands to extract data. However, these samples provide the flavor for how SQL is used.

Data Manipulation: Updating the Database

All of the examples involve queries to the database. Querying the database, however, is only one type of function that end-users need. End-users also need to change, add, and delete data from the database. Fortunately, SQL provides the facilities to perform these types of operations.

To add data to the database, the SQL command INSERT is used. In order to know where to insert the data, the DBMS needs to know both the table and the values that need to be inserted. Let's say that we want to insert a new patient in the patient table. This would be accomplished through the following command:

```
INSERT INTO PATIENT
    VALUES
    (7899999, "MCCOLLIGAN", "ELIZABETH", "A","F", 03-25-70)
```

What this command formulation says is to insert into the patient table the VALUES that follow. In this case, these are all the attributes of the patient table for a particular instance. This would result in the addition of a new record in the patient table for Elizabeth McColligan.

SQL provides the command UPDATE in order to change data in the database. Let's say that we want to change the middle initial for Frances Michaels. This would be accomplished by the UPDATE command followed by the name of the table in which the data are to be changed. After identifying the table, the attribute to be changed is identified. The following is a formulation of this operation:

```
UPDATE PATIENT
    SET MINITIAL = "P"
    WHERE MR# = 6789076
```

In the above example, the UPDATE command is followed by the name of the table. Then the attribute to be changed and the new value are identified. We also need to tell the DBMS what specific record needs to be updated. In this case, this was done by specifying the unique identifier, which is medical record number.

Many times data must be deleted. In SQL this is done through the DELETE command. Again, we must identify the table in which the data are to be deleted and also the specific record to be deleted. The following is an example of this formulation:

        DELETE PATIENT
            WHERE MR# = 7834561

Data Control

As discussed in Chapter 6, there are essentially two basic areas of data control. These include controlling access to the database and ensuring data integrity through transaction control. Since health information managers are more involved with data security and conceptual data modeling, the emphasis in this section is on access control commands.

As we learned in Chapter 6, database management systems provide functions whereby access to the database is controlled. Recall the authorization matrix in Chapter 6. This matrix describes the rights given to specific groups and/or individuals in regard to database access. For example, some employee groups may have access to certain data, but they cannot change or delete that data. Other employee groups may have more comprehensive rights to database access and control. The discussion that follows shows how the authorization matrix is operationalized using SQL.

The GRANT command is used to give specific employees or groups of employees access to, and privileges on, the database. The privileges that can be granted include the right to SELECT, UPDATE, ALTER, INSERT, and DELETE rows in the database tables. The SELECT command allows query of the database. The UPDATE command allows a user the privilege of changing attribute values in rows of the table. The ALTER command allows the user to add or delete columns (attributes) or to modify the data types of columns.

As we learned, the SELECT command allows user access to the database (i.e., to query the database). The SELECT function can be used to limit user access to certain columns (fields) and certain rows (records). For example, the admitting clerk should have access to only those data that are essential to performing the tasks assigned. Thus, access control would be accomplished through the following command:

        GRANT SELECT ON PATIENT
            TO ERTYUI, QWEDSA, . . .

The above command grants a query privilege to users ERTYUI and QWEDSA for all the columns in the PATIENT table. Note that ERTYUI and QWEDSA represent the user passwords of the individuals who are allowed to query the PATIENT table.

Another example of access control would be to extend to the admitting clerks privileges to update and to insert data in the PATIENT table. This would be accomplished by the following command:

    GRANT SELECT, UPDATE, INSERT ON PATIENT
        TO ERTYUI, QWEDSA

The result of this command is that the admitting clerks having the passwords ERTYUI and QWEDSA can query, change data, and add new patients to the PATIENT table.

If we would want to grant all privileges to an individual to the PATIENT table, the following command would be used:

    GRANT ALL ON PATIENT
        TO ZXCVBN

Certainly the above type of access with all privileges would be given to only a limited number of individuals.

Privileges that are given to individuals can be removed as well. For example, if an employee changes from one position to another in an organization, that employee's privileges to the database should also be changed. If an employee leaves the organization, then all privileges to the database should be removed immediately. The REVOKE command is used to remove some or all of an employee's privileges. The following command would be used to revoke all privileges for an employee:

    REVOKE ALL ON PATIENT
        FROM DFGVCX;

An example of a partial removal of privileges would be:

    REVOKE INSERT ON PATIENT
        FROM ERTYUI

The above command would revoke the insert (add) privilege to the admitting clerk with the password ERTYUI.

Access control also means creating user views or schemas. As we learned in Chapters 5 and 6, the conceptual model is an enterprise-wide view of the organization's data. The conceptual view is broken down into individual user views called subschemas. As Chapter 6 discusses, access to the database by employees is frequently limited to their user view or sub-schema. Thus, the end-user does not have access to everything in the database, but only to those data that are essential to performing the work task. For instance, say that we wanted to create a user view for a laboratory technician. Taking our ED example database, we would likely limit the laboratory technician view to the patient, encounter, and test/treatment tables. The columns that the technician would likely need access to in the patient table would include MR#, name, sex, and birthdate. In the encounter table the technician would likely need to know the date, and chief complaint. In the test/treatment table the technician would need to know test number, time ordered, time completed, and encounter number. In this case the CREATE command would be used as follows:

```
CREATE VIEW LABTECH
    SELECT MR#, NAME, SEX, BIRTHDATE, DATE, CHIEF COMPLAINT,
    TEST#, TIME_ORDERED, TIME_COMPLETE,
    FROM PATIENT, ENCOUNTER, TEST/TREATMENT
```

The learner can appreciate the importance of access control commands in regard to protecting the security of the database. These control commands or other variations on them would be used by the DA to grant and revoke privileges to end-users.

Conclusion

This discussion and examples provide a brief overview of SQL. Naturally there are many more SQL conventions and commands than those presented. Although SQL is a standard, some systems have "SQL-like" language. Therefore, SQL statements may vary from system to system. The examples here, however, provide a basic understanding of how such a query language functions in supporting end-user needs and maintenance of the database.

While SQL (and other such query languages) provides a mechanism to perform various operations on a database, the learner can see that the end-user must still be familiar with some basic programming logic and must be familiar with the database(s) being accessed. Therefore, this type of data manipulation language is not appropriate for every end-user to use. How, you might ask, does the end-user actually get access to the database to get routine work tasks done?

SQL statements can be embedded into a host language. The end-user does not see (or have to use) the SQL statements because they are already included in the program that is running the application. SQL statements can be included in computer programs that are written in third-generation programming languages such as COBOL, PL/1, or PASCAL. Recall that in Chapter 5 one of the criteria for a DBMS was that it support procedural languages such as COBOL and PASCAL. This feature is absolutely essential because it makes it possible for the application program to communicate with and manipulate the data in the relational database.

Embedding SQL statements in application programs takes care of routine tasks and applications. But what about ad hoc reports that may need to be created? For instance, what if the utilization management department wanted to retrieve data that were not included in regular, routine reports? SQL statements would need to be used to query the database and retrieve the necessary data. This is where the health information manager's expertise in SQL and knowledge of databases becomes valuable. By knowing the conceptual and subschema views of the database and having skill in a data manipulation language, the HIM can broker information to the end-user. In other words, the HIM can serve as an intermediary between the end-user and the database, retrieving data that are required on an ad hoc basis.

Query by Example

In addition to SQL, there is another popular data manipulation language called query by example (QBE). Whereas SQL and SQL-like languages are used in a mainframe environment, QBE is used principally in the microcomputer environment. Like SQL, there may be various versions of QBE. The differences among these versions, however, are minor. So once the HIM has skill in one QBE, it should be relatively easy to learn another version.

QBE is different from SQL because it frees the user from having to use structured statements and formats. QBE is used interactively on a display terminal and is supported today by easy-to-use graphic user interfaces (GUI). Although it depends on the QBE being used, the GUI will provide a space for the user to enter the name of the table to be queried. The QBE will automatically generate the names of the table columns. Figure 8-4. depicts such a screen from MicroSoft Access Database. Notice in this fig-

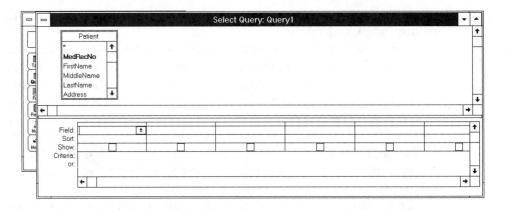

Figure 8-4.   QBE Screen with Attribute List

ure that the attributes (table columns) for the Patient file are listed in the window on the left of the screen.

Once this information is provided, the user indicates which columns are desired to be displayed. The system will then display the data for each of these columns. Figure 8-5 is an example of such a retrieval where the user had queried the database for a listing of patients' first and last name and city of residence.

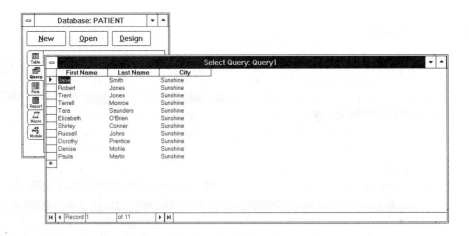

Figure 8-5.   QBE Screen with Attribute Data

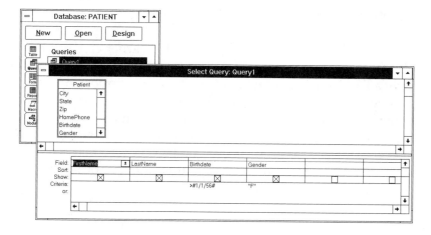

Figure 8-6.   QBE Screen with Conditional Query

Simple conditional queries are also easy to execute. Say we want to limit the retrievals to the patients who are female and whose date of birth is not earlier than 1956. In this case, we enter the value "F" in the GENDER column and the expression >1/1/56 in the BIRTHDATE column. Figure 8-6 shows this conditional query. Figure 8-7 shows the result of this query, which is a listing of only female patients who have a birthdate later than 1/1/56.

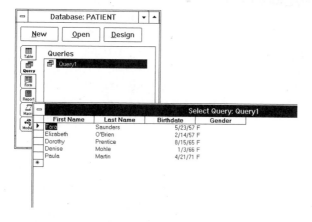

Figure 8-7.   QBE Conditional Query Result

The above QBE examples provide a brief overview of QBE. Tables can also be joined in QBE and other routine data definition and manipulation functions can be easily accomplished. As the learner can appreciate, QBE is a much more user-friendly interface than SQL. When evaluating and selecting a DBMS, as mentioned in Chapter 6, it is important that attention be given to the type of interface available to the end-user for ad hoc database query and manipulation. As the sample demonstrates, a GUI-based data manipulation language is much easier for end-users to use to generate their own ad hoc reports. Studies have indicated that the use of QBE produces similar or better results than other query approaches (Greenblat and Waxman, 1978).

Analyzing Data

To be useful, once data are retrieved they must be analyzed. The role of the HIM as a data analyst is becoming increasingly important. As more and more data are collected, there is a significant need to sift through these data and derive meaningful analysis. The methods discussed in this section are traditional methods of data analysis. The learner should be aware, however, that other methods using techniques such as neural networks, information filtering, and data mining are being developed in the computer and information sciences arena. These techniques use very large, complex data sets and mathematical algorithms to identify trends, make projections, and identify interesting relationships among data. These techniques are still in early stages of use. However, we would hope that the promise of such techniques will be realized in the near future. In the meantime, however, traditional data analysis methods are currently used in the health-care setting to assign meaning to data.

Analysis Design

The mere extraction of data is useless unless a reason for retrieval has been articulated. For example, the director of utilization management says, "Let me see a listing of the length of stay (LOS) of all patients treated within the past 6 months." The extraction of these data is virtually meaningless unless there is a reason for retrieval. The request would be better stated within the following context: "Let me see a listing of the LOS of all patients and their attending physicians so I can see if there is any relationship between LOS and physician." This statement makes a lot more sense because it provides a frame of reference for analysis. In this case, what the utilization management director is theorizing is that LOS is in some way related to certain physicians. Thus, the first step in any data analysis project is to specify the reason, theory, or hypothesis for which the data are being analyzed.

The second step in a data analysis project is to determine the variables that need to be gathered and analyzed. A variable is any characteristic or property that can be classified into two or more groups. For example, age can be classified by integers (1, 2, 3, 4). It can also be classified into ordinal groups such as infant, child, adolescent, and adult. Another example of a variable from the utilization management example is LOS. LOS can be classified into categories such as short or long. It can also be classified into integer data such as 1 day, 2 days, 3 days, and so on. From that same example, physician is another variable. It can be classified by specialty, say medicine, surgery, or pediatrics. Physician could also be classified by name as Dr. Smith, Dr. Jones, or Dr. Lyons. The variables that we choose for inclusion in a data analysis project should support our original reasons for studying a particular problem. For example, if we suspected that LOS was in some way related to physician utilization, then it would be meaningless to include zipcode as one of the characteristics we would want to analyze. However, if we suspected that there might be a relationship between LOS, physician, and the geographical location that a patient came from, then it would make sense to include zipcode in our study. When variables are selected for data analysis, they must support the questions we want to answer.

The third step in data analysis is the selection of the appropriate statistical procedures. Once the variables are selected, the data analyst can decide which statistical procedures will be best to answer the hypothesis or questions that are being studied. As we shall see later, the selection of variables becomes very important because some statistical procedures can only be used with certain types of scales of measurement.

Thus, the learner can see that data analysis should not be a "shooting from the hip" process. Developing an analysis plan is essential to obtaining good results. The better the planning is in hypothesis identification, variable selection, and statistical procedure choice, the better chance there is that results of the analysis will be meaningful and relevant.

Sample Case Data

To provide examples of various descriptive statistical methods, the data from a study of health-care chief information officers is used. Table 8-2 provides a description of the study and the type of data that were collected. This study was conducted to determine where CIOs worked, what their educational preparation had been, how many departments reported to them, how old they currently were, and what their gender was.

Fundamental Concepts

Levels of Measurement

One of the most fundamental concepts about data (variables) is level of measurement. Nominal, ordinal, interval, and ratio variables become very important in determining what statistical procedures can be used to analyze the data. For instance, some statistical procedures can only be performed using **interval data;** other statistical procedures are used exclusively with **nominal data.** Knowing what type of variables will be used in data collection will help the analyst determine what type of statistical tests can be used on that data.

Table 8-2.   CIO Survey Study

Sample:	250 Health-Care Chief Information Officers	
Response Rate:	60%	
Variables Collected:	Hospital Size	Interval Data
	Type of Facility	Nominal Data
	Level of CIO Position	Nominal Data
	Number of Departments Reporting to CIO	Ratio Data
	Functions Reporting to CIO	Nominal Data
	Educational Degree	Nominal Data
	Years in Current Position	Ratio Data
	Gender	Nominal Data
	Age	Ratio Data

Nominal variables have positively defined categories with no implied distance between one category and the next. Gender, marital status, mode of arrival at the hospital, and medical specialty would all be examples of nominal variables. In the CIO study, notice how many of the variables are nominal data. Each of these categories is mutually exclusive and there is no implied equal distance among them.

Ordinal variables belong to categories and these categories can be ordered or ranked. The amount of difference or distance between these categories, however, may not be equal. Common ordinal variables are social class (i.e., upper, middle, and lower class) and categories such as strongly disagree, disagree, agree, and strongly agree.

Variables that are numeric are called interval and ratio variables. These variables have the characteristics of nominal and ordinal variables (i.e., they can be categorized and ranked), but they also can be defined in terms of a standard unit of measurement. In other words, the distance between points has a real meaning. An example of an interval variable is temperature reading. Unlike interval data, ratio data have a true zero point. Examples of ratio data include age, hematocrit count, and white blood cell count. The important thing about interval and ratio data is that they can be manipulated arithmetically by addition and subtraction; averages can be calculated and other sophisticated statistical techniques can be performed.

Discrete and Continuous Data

Interval data (numerical) can be either **discrete** or **continuous.** Data are said to be discrete when they are plotted on a number scale and they lie only on certain points and not on the points in between. Continuous data, on the other hand, can theoretically lie anywhere within a specified interval on a number scale. For example, if we were counting how many patients had received physical therapy treatment on an outpatient basis during the month of March, the result would be a count of individuals. These data would be discrete. The result of our counting would be a number that could lie only on certain number points. In this case, it would be a whole number, since half of a patient could not receive a physical therapy treatment. An example of a continuous data set would be the temperature readings of a patient. In this case, any value between relevant points could be possible. Figure 8-8 shows how discrete and continuous data would be represented on a number scale.

Discrete Data Set

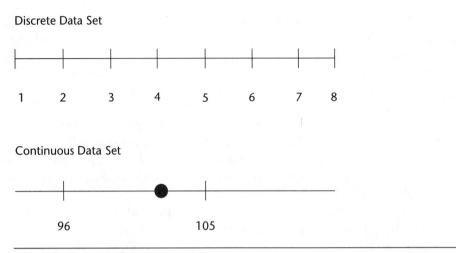

Continuous Data Set

Figure 8-8. Discrete and Continuous Data Examples

The top line shows that data points can fall only on certain points on the line—1, 2, 3, 4, 5, 6, 7, and 8. This line would fit our physical therapy example, where we could only have whole numbers of people who had received therapy. The bottom line shows that data can lie on any point between 96 and 105. This line would fit our temperature example, since a patient's temperature could fall anywhere within that interval. In the CIO study example there are several continuous variables, including age and years in current position.

Descriptive Measures

Data can be summarized in a variety of ways. This summarization is often referred to as descriptive statistics. Summarization of data includes counting frequencies, determining the **mean, median,** and **mode** (measures of central tendency) and calculating the **variance** and **standard deviation** (measures of dispersion). The calculation of descriptive statistics is usually the first step in analyzing data.

Frequency Distribution

One way of summarizing a data set is by **frequency distribution.** The range of all values is divided into ordered classes and the number of observations that falls into each class is determined. A frequency distribution can be done with nominal, ordinal, interval, and ratio data. A good example of frequency distribution from the CIO study is the frequency of how many years a CIO has been in his or her current position. This distribution is depicted in Table 8-3. To interpret this table, we can see that 23 out of 139 CIOs have been in their positions for 1 year, 25 out of 139 CIOs have been in their positions for 2 years, and so on. Notice that a percent frequency and cumulative percent are also provided in this table. A frequency distribution provides a good picture of the pattern or distribution of observations. This is especially the case when both the raw frequencies and a percentage frequency is provided such as in Table 8-3. What we can tell from this table is that most CIOs are in their current position for not more than 5 years. We could say that after 5 years in a job position, the longevity of the CIO rapidly declines.

Table 8-3.   Frequency Distribution of Longevity in Current CIO Position

Years	*Frequency*	*Percent*	*Cumulative Percent*
1	23	16.5	16.5
2	25	18.0	34.5
3	26	18.7	53.2
4	12	8.6	61.8
5	16	11.5	73.3
6	12	8.6	81.9
7	4	3.0	84.9
8	4	3.0	87.9
9	1	.7	88.6
10	8	5.8	94.4
11	1	.7	95.1
12	1	.7	95.8
13	1	.7	96.5
16	1	.7	96.2
19	1	.7	97.9
20	1	.7	98.6
24	1	.7	99.3
35	1	.7	100
Total	139		

Measures of Central Tendency

Even though a frequency distribution provides a good picture of a trend, other summarization is needed to fully describe a data set. The most popular measures to summarize data are called **measures of central tendency.** They include the mean, median, and mode. They indicate the "typical" value of a variable, for example, the mean is the average of set of values. To calculate the mean, the values of the variable for each case are added and then divided by that number of cases. Only interval or ratio data can be used to calculate the mean. In the CIO example, the mean or average number of years in current position is 4.7 years.

Although the mean is a good measure for interval data, it cannot be used with ordinal or nominal data. The alternative measure for **ordinal data** is the median, and the alternative measure for nominal or ordinal data is the mode. (Both median and mode, however, can also be used with interval data.)

What is the median? The median is the midpoint number in a frequency distribution. In order to calculate the median, the data set must first be put in ranking order from lowest to highest value. After the data set is put in order, the middle number or observation is identified. Technically the median value should have half of the remaining values above it and the other half below it. Looking at our CIO example again, the total number of cases is 139. The middle observation would be 70 (i.e., 69 observations above and 69 observations below). Now looking at Table 8-3, we can figure out the median number of years that CIOs have been in their current position. To find the median observation, we simply add the frequencies until we get to the 70th observation. In this case, we add 23 observations (1 year) + 25 observations (2 years) + 26 observations (3 years) = 74. Since 70 is our median observation, it falls within the 3-year category. Thus, we can say that the median length of time a CIO has spent in the current position is 3 years. Note that the median in this case is quite a bit smaller than the average, which is 4.7 years.

The mode is the most frequently occurring category or the most frequently occurring number in a set of observations. The mode can be used with interval, ordinal, or nominal data. The modal length of longevity of a CIO is 3 years—that is, the 3-year category is the category that most frequently occurs.

To summarize our findings of central tendency for the CIO data set, we now know that the average length of longevity in the current position is

4.7 years, the median is 3 years, and the mode is 3 years. From these findings it is important to calculate all measures of central tendency if possible. In this case, the mean number 4.7 is significantly higher than the median and mode, because the mean can be unduly influenced by a few extreme values. If we look at the frequency distribution in Table 8-3, we can see that there are a number of extreme values that cause the mean to be higher than the median and mode. Ideally we would like to see all three measures of central tendency for the same data set. Because the measures are quite a bit different among the mean, median, and mode, we will want to be careful in reporting these data. What we should do is report at least the mean and the median. Do not be satisfied with data only about the mean. Require that additional measures of central tendency be reported as well.

Measures of Dispersion

Measures of dispersion or **variance** provide yet another perspective for describing a data set. Measures of dispersion provide data about the spread among the individual observations. Different groups of observations may have the same mean, median, and mode yet may differ widely with respect to the spread among the individual observations. The range, standard deviation, and variance are measures of dispersion.

The range of a data set is the difference between the largest and smallest values. In the CIO example, the range in time in position is 34 years (35 years – 1 year). The reporting of the range of values does not provide us with too much information. All we know is that the range is fairly large for this data set, but it does not tell us how the observations were distributed within this range. However, when taken into account with the frequency distribution, the range helps us to get a better picture of the data.

Another measure of dispersion is the variance. What we are trying to determine with the variance is how dispersed the cases are from the mean. The variance is an average deviation of the difference between the mean and each of the individual values in the data set. In other words, do most of the cases cluster close to the mean? If the variance is zero, then we know that all the scores have the same value. The smaller the variance, the closer the cases are to the mean; the larger the variance, the more widely the cases are scattered. We do not have to be concerned here with how the variance is calculated. The details of calculation should be left to a course in statistics. What is important is that the variance is used as a foundation for calculating other vital statistical measures. The variance for the CIO data in Table 8-3 is 21.

The variance by itself, however, does not tell us too much. A statistical measure based on the variance that helps us visualize the data better is the standard deviation. The standard deviation is based on the premise of a normal distribution of values. A normal distribution is represented in Figure 8-9

As Figure 8-9 shows, for any normal distribution, approximately 68 percent of the cases will fall within +1 to –1 standard deviations from the mean; approximately 95 percent of the cases will fall within +2 to –2 standard deviations from the mean and 99 percent of the cases will fall within +3 to –3 standard deviations from the mean. Thus, if we know the standard deviation, we can visualize not only how dispersed the cases are away from the mean but we can also determine whether or not our observations are normally distributed. The notion of normal distribution becomes very important because the utility of a standard deviation is based on the use of data that form a normal distribution. If you do not have a normal distribution of data, calculation of the standard deviation

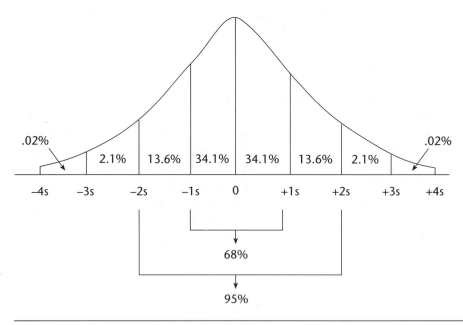

Figure 8-9.   Normal Population Distribution

and other advanced statistical measures becomes less reliable. An example is provided later with the CIO data.

The closer the standard deviation is to zero, the less variance there is among the cases. Let's take a hypothetical case to look at mean, variance, and standard deviation interpretations. Assume we are studying the LOS for patients with GOK (God only knows) disease. The frequency distribution is presented in Table 8-4.

The range of LOS is 8 days (9 days – 1 day). The mean LOS is 5 days and the median and mode in this case is also 5 days. These data begin to indicate that the data are fairly evenly dispersed. However, we want to get another perspective about the actual dispersion among the data. We calculate the variance and standard deviation. (Don't concern yourself with how these numbers are calculated.) The variance in this case is 2.5 and the standard deviation is 1.6. The standard deviation tells us that we would expect 68 percent of our cases to be between an LOS of 3.4 and 6.6 days (i.e., +1 to –1 standard deviations from the mean); that 95 percent of our cases would be between an LOS of 1.8 and 8.2 days (i.e., +2 to –2 standard deviations from the mean); and that 99 percent of our cases would be between an LOS of .2 and 9.8 days (i.e., +3 to –3 standard deviations of the mean). Figure 8-10 shows the mean of our data with the standard deviations.

Table 8-4. Frequency Distribution of LOS for Patients with GOK Disease

Days	Frequency	Percent	Cumulative Percent
1	1	2.9	2.9
2	1	2.9	5.8
3	3	8.5	14.4
4	5	14.3	28.6
5	15	42.8	71.4
6	5	14.3	85.7
7	3	8.5	94.2
8	1	2.9	97.1
9	1	2.9	100

Total   35

Mean = 5

Variance = 2.5

Standard Deviation = 1.69

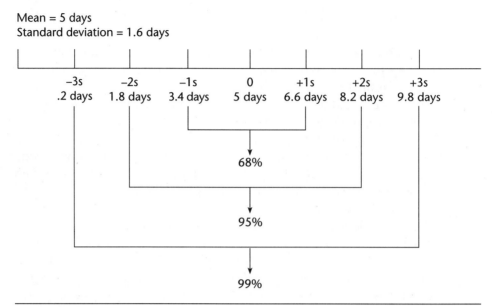

Mean = 5 days
Standard deviation = 1.6 days

| −3s | −2s | −1s | 0 | +1s | +2s | +3s |
| .2 days | 1.8 days | 3.4 days | 5 days | 6.6 days | 8.2 days | 9.8 days |

68%

95%

99%

Figure 8-10. LOS Mean and Standard Deviations

Now we need to determine whether or not our data set approximates a normal distribution. We know that we have 35 cases total. If we have an approximate normal distribution, we would expect that 68 percent of the 35 cases (24 cases) would be between 3.4 and 6.6 days. An inspection of the frequency distribution in Table 8-4 shows that there are 25 cases within this range. We would also expect that 95 percent of the 35 cases (33 cases) would have an LOS between 1.8 and 8.2 days. As we can see from the frequency table there are 33 cases within this range. Thus, from these data we can feel comfortable that the data set essentially represents a normal distribution of data and is well described by the mean and standard deviation.

If a data set does not closely approximate the normal distribution, then the mean and standard deviation are not good descriptors of the data. Our CIO data are a case in point. With the CIO data, recall that the mean is 4.7 years and the median and mode are 3 years. The variance for the CIO data is 21 and the standard deviation is 4.6. If we were to plot out the years in current position on a line graph, we would expect 68 percent of the CIOs to be in their current positions between .76 and 9.1 years. Since there are 139 cases, 68 percent of these would be 94 cases. Inspection of the CIO frequency distribution in Table 8-3, however, shows that 122 cases fall within this range.

Clearly these data are not normally distributed. Thus, the mean and standard deviation are not good descriptors of these data. If this is the case, how do we go about analyzing the data? Fortunately, there are alternatives!

As you already know, the median and mode are useful descriptors of data. When we have data that are not normally distributed, the mean, median, and mode should all be reported. These data taken together provide a better picture of the dispersion of data and whether or not there are extreme values that may be unduly influencing the calculation of the mean.

In regard to an alternative to the standard deviation, the calculation of percentiles is usually preferred when the data are not normally distributed. A percentile is a number that divides a distribution into 100 equal parts. Thus, if a value is said to be in the 10th percentile, it means that 10 percent of all the values in the data set are below this value. The percentile calculation is based on the median. It is not influenced like the mean by extreme scores in either direction. The percentiles for the CIO data are reported in Table 8-3. Notice that while the mean is 4.7 years, the 50th percentile is 3 years. If we were to report only that the average years in the current position of a CIO is 4.7 years, this would be misleading—the mean is 4.7, *but* 50 percent of CIOs have been in their current position for only 3 years. Thus, the percentile is a better descriptor of the years in current CIO position.

As this discussion demonstrates, data analysts should not rely on only one measure for description of the data. It is essential that all measures be included for analysis, and based on this analysis, the measures that best describe the data should be reported.

Measures of Association

Providing a description of data is frequently not enough to answer questions that may be of interest. More often than not, the reason for performing a data analysis is to determine if there is a relationship between two or more variables. In the example of LOS for GOK disease, perhaps the real question for study is whether or not there is a relationship between specific patients and LOS. Or perhaps the question is whether or not there is a relationship between LOS and attending physician. To answer these questions, statistical procedures that measure associations are required. Measures of association are often referred to as correlation coefficients.

Measures of association are calculated to summarize the degree of relationship between a pair of variables. Variable association means that a change in one variable is accompanied by a change in another variable. If two variables change together, then we say that they are associated or related. For example, if the LOS of a patient increases, as the age of the patient increases, then we would say that there is an association between the variables LOS and age. This would be a positive correlation.

When we talk about two or more variables, it is necessary to distinguish between dependent and independent variables. The dependent variable is the variable that we wish to explain something about. The independent variables are other variables used in explaining the behavior of the dependent variable. In the example of LOS and age, LOS would be the dependent variable (the variable that we wish to explain) and age would be an independent variable (used in explaining why LOS changes).

Variables can have either a positive or a negative relationship. A positive relationship is one in which an increase in the independent variable is accompanied by an increase in the dependent variable. The LOS and age example is an example of a positive relationship. As age (the independent variable) increases, it is accompanied by the increase in LOS (the dependent variable). Relationships between variables can also be negative—an increase in the independent variable is accompanied by a decrease in the dependent variable. For example, an increase in the dosage of a beta blocker (independent variable) is accompanied by a decrease in heartbeat (dependent variable). There is no relationship between variables when the dependent variable is as likely to increase, decrease, or remain the same when the independent variable changes.

Statistical tests used to determine measures of association are designed to indicate how strong the relationship is and whether the relationship is positive or negative. For example, the Pearson R is usually reported as –1.0 to 1.0. If the measure equals 0.0, then there is no relationship. If the measure is greater than 0, then it is a positive relationship. If the measure is less than 0, then the relationship is negative. The closer the measure is to either 1.0 or –1.0, the stronger the relationship. Thus, a relationship of +.89 is stronger than a relationship of +.25 in the positive direction. Similarly, a relationship of –.89 is stronger than a relationship of –.25 in the negative direction.

It is important to understand that there are many different measures or tests that can be done to determine variable association. The type of test performed will depend on whether or not the variables are nominal, ordinal, or interval. A test designed for interval data cannot be used when the data are nominal. Therefore, when the study design is developed, it is

Table 8-5.   Measures of Association

Variable Type	Measures of Association	Values
Nominal Variables	Lambda	0.0 to +1.0
	Goodman & Kruskal's tau-*y*	0.0 to +1.0
Ordinal Variables	Kendall's tau-*a*	−1.0 to +1.0
	Gamma (G)	−1.0 to + 1.0
	Sommers' *d*	−1.0 to +1.0
	Tau-*b*	−1.0 to +1.0
	Spearman's rho (r_s)	−1.0 to +1.0
Interval Variables	Pearson's product-moment correlation coefficient, *r*	−1.0 to +1.0
	Coefficient of determination, r^2	0 to 1

important to identify the level of the variables in order to determine the statistical test that can be performed on the data. Common measures of association are reported in Table 8-5.

Each of the statistical tests has certain conventions that must be followed. These tests are also used to measure different types of associations. For example, lambda is concerned with predicting an optimal value that is the mode of the dependent variable, whereas tau-*y* predicts the distribution of the dependent variable. Thus, the choice of test to determine the association between variables not only depends on the variable type (nominal, ordinal, or interval) but also on the type of explanation desired.

So far we have only discussed associations between one dependent and one independent variable. What happens when we want to look at associations between more than two variables? For example, what if we want to determine if there is a relationship between LOS and two independent variables such as age and income? A test that measures the association of many independent variables with a dependent variable is multiple regression. The multiple correlation coefficient is represented by *R* and its square by R^2.

For the purposes of this text, it is not important to delve into all the various mathematical explanations and theory. What is important, however, is for the HIM to understand that correct statistical tests must be applied so that data are analyzed appropriately. The HIM should also be able to critically assess whether or not analysis done by others has been appropriately carried out.

Determining Significance and Group Differences

Often the data analyst wants to determine whether or not a certain result is statistically significant. There are many sophisticated definitions of **statistical significance.** For our purposes, however, we will say that when we try to determine whether or not a result is statistically significant we are trying to determine whether or not the result is due to chance. We want to know whether the result we obtained from our sample occurred by chance or whether it is truly reflective of the population from which we drew our sample. For instance, let's say that we were looking at whether or not following a certain drug regimen for a given condition had an effect on lowering patient morbidity. Perhaps we had 1,000 of these types of cases in our facility over the past 5 years. Rather than reviewing all 1,000 cases, we took a random sample of 100 cases to review. Our analysis indicated that indeed there was a relationship between protocol use and the reduction of the patient morbidity. But how can we be sure that result is not a function of chance and that it truly represents the total population of 1,000 cases? The answer to determine whether or not this result really reflects the population of all the cases is to perform a test of significance. Too frequently in health-care facility studies, samples are drawn from a larger population, but tests of significance are never done. The HIM analyst must be sensitive to this problem.

There are many types of tests of significance. In this section we explain a few of the more popular ones. Just as tests of association depend on whether or not the variables under study are nominal, ordinal, or interval, so too do tests of significance depend on this—the right test must be applied to the right type of data. A test used to determine significance of interval data cannot be used on data that are nominal. For nominal data, one of the most popular tests of significance is the chi-square test (X^2). Other tests of significance for ordinal and interval data include the t-test and F-statistic.

The t-test is a test of significance that is used when we are trying to determine whether or not means of two groups on one variable are statistically different from each other. This is called a univariate (meaning one variable) test of significance. For instance, say that we were studying the white blood cell counts (WBC) of a group of patients that had a specific condition. Say that we took a sample of 100 cases from the total patient population of 5,000 cases. We then calculated the mean WBC count for our sample and found that the mean was 10,000. What we really would want to know is whether or not this mean is the same as that for the total population of patients. We would apply a mathematical formula that would calculate the *t*-test. From the result of the *t*-test we could then determine whether or not the mean of the WBC count in our sample was the same as that of the total population—that is, statistically significant.

T-tests are also used to determine if there is a difference between the means of two groups. Let's say that we are doing a study that looks at the difference between health-care utilization between two different groups of people—people who belong to health maintenance organizations (HMOs) and people who do no not belong to HMOs. Assume that health-care utilization is being defined as charges for service. We want to discover if means for charges of service for these groups are significantly different from each other. We would take a random sample of 100 from the group of HMO members and 100 from the group who were not HMO members. We would calculate the mean charge for each group. Let's say the HMO group mean charge for the year was $467 and the mean charge for the non-HMO group was $425. We want to find out whether or not this is a true difference between the groups (and is representative of the means for the total population) or whether this difference is a function of chance. Since we have the means for each group, we can apply the mathematical formula for a two-group *t*-test and get the *t*-statistic. We can then determine whether or not the difference between the two groups is statistically significant.

What do we do when we want to study more than two groups? For example, let's say that we wanted to see if there was a difference between the means of three groups of patients: group A, group B, and group C. Suppose each group was on a different type of therapy for a certain condition and that we were using their hematocrit levels as a measure for their condition. A higher hematocrit indicates a better response to the therapy. Let's say that group A had a hematocrit mean of 42, group B had a hematocrit mean of 45, and group C had a hematocrit mean of 38. To determine whether or not there is a statistical difference between these means we would apply a mathematical formula to calculate an *F*-statistic. This type of test is called an analysis of variance (ANOVA). From this test and its associated *F*-statistic we could then determine whether or not the differences between group means were statistically significant. If the means were significantly different, we might want to infer that the treatment used with group B produced a better result than the treatments used for group A and group C.

What happens when we want to look at the effect of two or more independent variables on a dependent variable? This procedure is called multivariate (more than one variable) tests of significance. To determine if there are differences between two or more independent variables we can use statistical tests such as multivariate analysis of variance (MANOVA) or multiple regression.

It is important to learn from this section that appropriate statistical tests must be used to analyze data. Too frequently the analyst is not familiar with the purpose or application of these tests and results of analysis are limited to descriptive procedures.

Data Presentation Techniques

An important part of data analysis is the method of data presentation. There are a variety of methods and techniques for presenting data. Some of these techniques are suited for certain types of data. For example, you would not want to use a line graph with nominal data. Therefore, presentation techniques must be used correctly if the meaning of data are to be represented appropriately. Some years ago a delightful book called *How to Lie with Statistics* (1954) was published. This book presented a number of ways in which data presentation techniques could be used to misrepresent the meaning of data. It usually is not the intent of the data analyst to intentionally deceive others about the results of analysis. However, unintentional deception is often the case when the analyst does not know the principles of appropriate data presentation. The intent of this section is to provide an overview of some of the principles associated with graphing so the data analyst can use techniques appropriately and critique the data presentation of others.

Graphing Data

An important aim for any data analyst is to highlight the information contained in data so that clinicians, providers, executives, and others can examine it and draw appropriate conclusions. Representation of data through the use of graphs has much to offer when complex relationships must to be clarified.

Histograms, polygons, and **line graphs** are basic graphical procedures. Basic to understanding any graphical technique is the idea of a reference system or coordinate system. The usual coordinate system for graphing includes lines drawn at right angles to each other. This is called the Cartesian coordinate system. Figure 8-11 depicts a two-dimension Cartesian coordinate reference system. The vertical line is called the Y axis

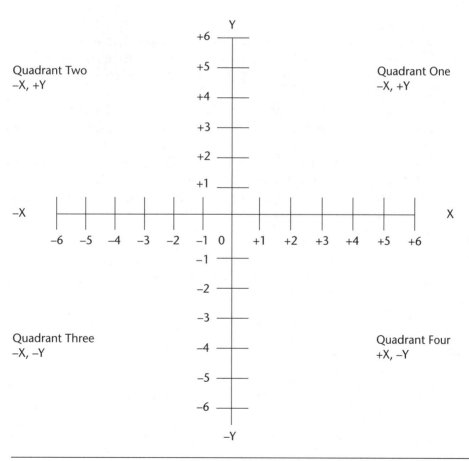

Figure 8-11. Cartesian Coordinate System

or ordinate. The horizontal line is called the X axis or abscissa. These lines divide the plane into four quadrants. The zero point on both axes is the point where the axes cross. All number systems extend outward from the zero point. The scores going upward from the zero point on the Y axis are positive scores. The scores going down from the zero point on the Y axis are negative scores. Scores to the right of the zero point on the X axis are positive scores and scores to the left of the zero point on the X axis are negative scores. Since most data that are examined in a health-care organization are positive, quadrant one is the graphical picture we see most often.

Histogram

A histogram is a plot of frequency or percentage distribution. The frequency or percentage is plotted on the Y axis. The X and Y axes always begin at the point of origin (i.e., zero). This is done so that distortions in data presentation are avoided. The X axis score may begin with zero or any convenient low score.

Table 8-6 depicts a frequency distribution of CIOs in various size hospitals. We can see that this distribution reports frequency, percent, and cumulative percent. In order to get a different perspective of the data, a histogram can be used. Figure 8-12 is a frequency histogram and Figure 8-13 represents a percentage histogram. Note that the Y axis of each histogram begins at zero. Note that in Figure 8-12 the symbol f is used at the top of the Y axis to indicate that this is a frequency histogram. Note that in

Table 8-6.   Frequency Distribution of CIOs by Hospital Bed Size

Bed Size	Frequency	Percent	Cumulative Percent
200	7	5.1	5.1
300	14	10.1	15.2
400	24	17.4	32.6
500	23	16.7	49.3
600	30	21.7	71
700	20	14.6	85.6
800	10	7.2	92.8
900	5	3.6	96.4
1000	5	3.6	100
Total	138		

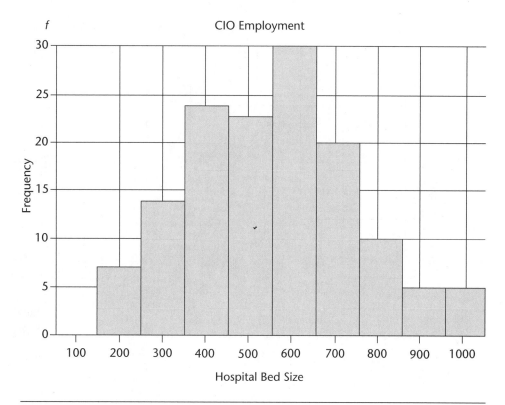

Figure 8-12. Frequency Histogram: CIOs by Hospital Bed Size

Figure 8-13 the symbol % is used to indicate that this is a percentage frequency. Note also that in each graph regular intervals are used on the Y axis—5, 10, 15, 20, 25. The height of the Y axis corresponds to somewhat more than the maximum frequency. The Y axis should always be at least three-fourths of, or equal to, the length of the X axis.

Note that the variable for the X axis is clearly marked as "hospital bed size." The rectangles are constructed to a height that represents the frequency for a given category. The sides of each rectangle come down at the exact category boundaries. The data represented in this example are discrete, interval data. A logical question to pose is whether or not histograms can be used for ordinal or nominal data. Histograms are also used to graph ordinal data. However, when nominal data are used, the graph that is used is referred to as a **bar chart.** Figure 8-14 (page 249) is an example of a

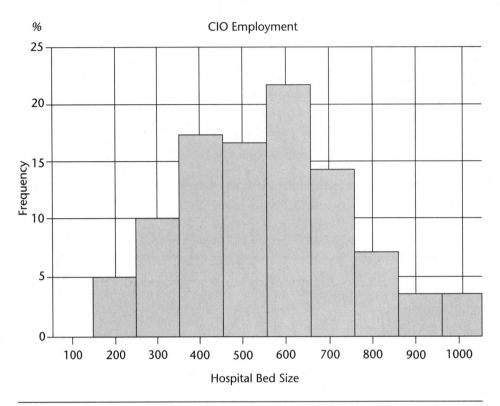

Figure 8-13.   Percentage Histogram

bar chart or bar graph. Note that when nominal data are used, the bars are separated somewhat to indicate that these categories are separate and distinct from each other. In Figure 8-14 we see the frequency of males and females depicted for a certain condition.

Frequency Polygons

A polygon is a graph that also represents frequencies and percentages. A polygon is a figure that connects frequency points plotted on the Y axis with points plotted above the midpoint of the category on the X axis. Using the CIO data from the above example, Figures 8-15 (page 250) and 8-16 (page 251) represent frequency and percentage polygons. Polygons are particularly useful in graphing interval data because the visual impression that

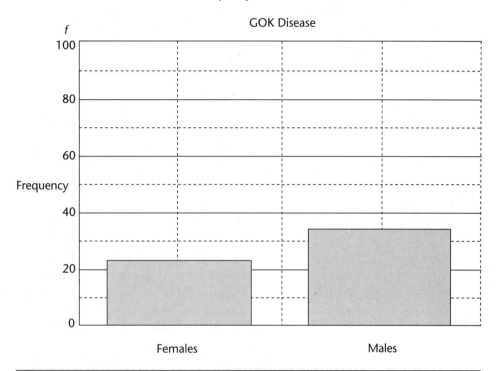

Figure 8-14.   Bar Chart

is presented is of more gradual shifts in frequency or percentage from category to category

Polygons and histograms can be used to distinguish differences in frequencies and percentages between groups. Figure 8-17 shows two groups of patients. Group A received an antibiotic and group B did not receive an antibiotic. The graphs in Figure 8-17 (page 252) show the comparisons of the two WBC count distributions between those patients who received the antibiotic and those who did not.

Line Graphs

Another type of graph is the line graph. The line graph displays the value of the dependent variable (represented on the Y axis) for each of several

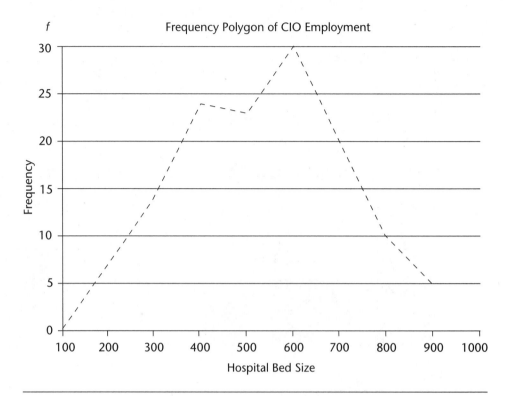

Figure 8-15. Frequency Polygon

categories on an independent variable (represented on the X axis). Notice that in a line graph we are trying to represent relationships among data, whereas with the histogram and polygon, frequency distributions were being represented.

Figure 8-18 (page 252) is a line graph using hypothetical data about the relationship of patient age (independent variable) and the number of clinic visits made per year (dependent variable). Note that in this figure each axis is clearly marked with the names of the variables under study.

Distortions in Graphing

Whatever type of graphical technique is used, it is important that sound construction principles are followed. To communicate the data clearly,

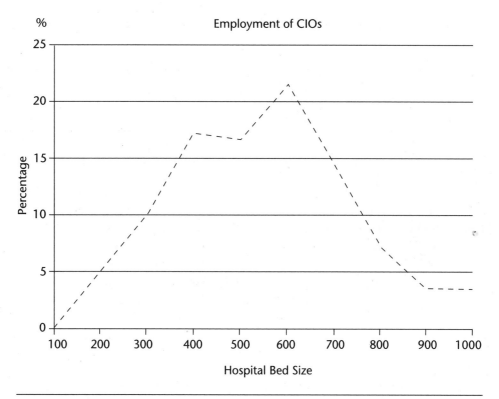

Figure 8-16. Percentage Polygon

knowledge about what is to be communicated is required as well as what potential misinterpretations could occur. Some examples of how data can be distorted through the use of graphs include:

- Shortening the Y or X axis. Remember that the Y axis should always be three-fourths to equally as long as the X axis.
- Not starting with zero on the frequency or percentage scale of the Y axis for histograms or polygrams.
- Use of figures that differ in volume or size.

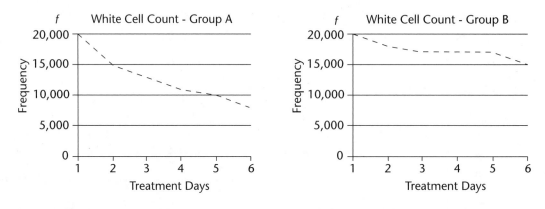

Figure 8-17. Comparison between Two Groups Using Polygons

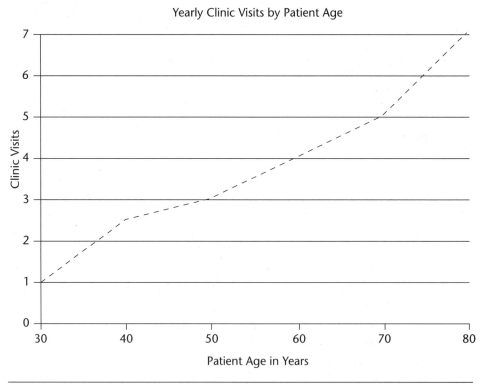

Figure 8-18. Line Graph Comparing Independent and Dependent Variable

Use of Computer Statistical Packages

In the 1990s, the availability of software packages for statistical computation has increased enormously. These packages, such as the Statistical Package for the Social Sciences (SPSS), are now available with GUI interfaces that the end-user can use almost intuitively to perform a variety of statistical tests. Most of these software packages are available for microcomputers and interface easily to a variety of database systems. The packages not only perform statistical calculations but have graphing capabilities as well. The HIM should have a working knowledge and skill of at least one of these statistical packages.

Summary

- Data retrieval and analysis are two important domains of practice of the health information manager.
- The primary way data are retrieved and manipulated in a database is through the use of a data manipulation language (DML). Two of the more popular DMLs are structured query language (SQL) and query by example (QBE).
- A DML usually contains commands for data definition, manipulation, and control. Data definition allows for the creation of database tables and definition of attributes. Data manipulation allows for query and change to the database. Data control restricts access to the database.
- The design of any data analysis project involves three basic steps: (1) identifying the questions or reason for study, (2) determining the variables of interest, and (3) selecting appropriate statistical procedures for data analysis.
- A variable can have either a nominal, ordinal, or interval level of measurement.
- Summarization of data is referred to as descriptive statistics. Frequency distributions, measures of central tendency, and measures of dispersion are techniques for summarizing data.
- Measures of central tendency include the mean, median, and mode. Measures of dispersion include the variance and standard deviation.

- Measures of association are calculated to summarize the degree of relationship or association between a pair of variables. The type of measure of association used depends on the level of measurement of the variable. Common measures of association for nominal data include lambda and tau-y. A popular measure for association for ordinal data is Spearman's rho and popular measures for association for interval data are Pearson's product moment correlation coefficient (r) and coefficient determinant r^2.

- Tests of significance are performed to determine whether or not the mean of a sample truly represents the population mean. Univariate tests of significance are used to study the effects of one variable on one or two groups. Multivariate tests of significance are used to study the effects of two or more variables on one or more groups. Popular tests of significance include the t-test, analysis of variance (ANOVA), and mutivariate analysis of variance (MANOVA).

Review Questions

1. Discuss why the role of data retrieval and analysis is important in today's health-care environment.

2. Discuss the obstacles that exist in data retrieval. How can these be overcome?

3. Compare the features and functions of SQL and QBE. What are the strengths and weakness of each?

4. Describe the steps that should be included in designing a data analysis project. What happens if one of these steps is not included in the design phase of the project?

5. Discuss the concept of levels of measurement. Why is knowing the level of measurement of a variable important?

6. Distinguish between various data descriptive measures. Discuss when it is appropriate (or inappropriate) to use each of these measures. What additional perspectives do each of these measures bring to the analysis of data?

7. Explain what is meant by a measure of association. What are the various measures of association?

8. Explain what is meant by statistical significance. Why are tests of statistical significance performed? What are some tests of statistical significance?

9. Discuss the differences between histograms, polygons, line graphs, and bar charts. When and with what type of data are these tests appropriate to use?

10. Discuss ways that data can be distorted through errors in data graphing.

Enrichment Activities

1. Obtain several examples of data analysis from several local health-care facilities. For each analysis, describe its strengths and weaknesses. For example, were the correct statistical tests and measures applied? Should additional statistical tests have been done? If the data are graphically represented, are there any flaws in the presentation? What corrective measures would you suggest?

2. Review examples of data analysis from articles in health information management journals. Are the analyses appropriate? Should additional analyses have been done? Given the data analysis in the article(s), how confident are you of the results?

References

Greenblat, D., and Waxman, J. (1978). A study of three database query languages. In *Databases: Improving Usability and Responsiveness*, B. Schneideman, (ed.). New York: Academic Press.

Huff, D. (1954). *How to Lie with Statistics.* New York: W.W. Norton & Co.

Chapter 9

Security, Audit, and Control of Health Data

Learning Objectives

After completing this chapter, the learner should be able to:

1. Discuss the imperatives for development of national legislation that addresses issues of informational privacy.
2. Discuss the dimensions of data security and why these are important to the development of a total security program.
3. Address how the goals of a data security program should be implemented and managed in a health-care enterprise.
4. Conduct a risk assessment and analysis for a given information system application.
5. Given the results of a risk assessment and analysis, recommend appropriate security countermeasures.
6. Given the results of a risk assessment and analysis, develop an appropriate business continuity plan for a given information systems application.

Key Terms

Annualized Loss Expectancy
Business Continuity Plan

Chief Security Officer

Computer-Based Patient Record

Computer-Based Patient Record Institute

Confidentiality

Electronic Data Interchange

Privacy

Risk Analysis

Risk Assessment

Trojan Horse

Worm

Introduction

Security, audit, and control of patient-related health data is a critical component in all health-care information systems. While methods for ensuring data security are practiced in other industries, the underlying philosophy for data protection in the health-care arena is fundamentally different. In industries outside of health care, the primary focus of a data security program is to ensure that sensitive information is made available only to authorized individuals in order to protect the interests of the organization. In health care, protection of organizational interests is secondary to the protection of the interests and rights of the patient. Thus, any health-care data security program must be grounded in a fundamental philosophy of recognizing an individual's right to privacy and to maintaining the confidentiality of the physician–patient relationship.

As health care moves toward more automation of data and the development of the computer-based patient record, it is imperative that data security, audit, and control techniques be made an integral part of the planning and implementation of enterprise, regional, and national health information system infrastructures. Data security, audit, and control methods are not the only issues pertaining to the safekeeping of information. There are other factors connected with the control of data, such as goals to ensure that data are accurate, correct, reliable, and complete. Issues relating to data quality are addressed in previous chapters. This chapter focuses on methods and techniques for ensuring that individual privacy and information confidentiality concerns are adequately addressed as well as systematically incorporated into the development of the health information infrastructure.

Privacy and Confidentiality of Health Data

Confidentiality and **privacy** are concepts associated with the rights of patients. Frequently there is a misconception about the meaning of these terms and sometimes they are misused or interchanged. Privacy is usually understood to mean the right of an individual to limit access by others to some aspect of their person. In the case of health data, the focus is on informational privacy (Gostin et al., 1995). Informational privacy includes the right of an individual to determine at what time, in what way, and to what extent information about him or her is communicated to others. An example of informational privacy is when a patient freely shares personal information with a physician or other health practitioner. Confidentiality, on the other hand, is based on a special doctor–patient relationship and "refers to the expectation that the information collected will be used for the purpose for which it was gathered" (Bialorucki and Blane, 1992). In the case of confidentiality, the patient has the expectation that information shared with a health-care provider will be used for its intended purpose (diagnosis and treatment) and that this information will not be disclosed to others unless the patient is first made aware and consents to its disclosure. Due to issues of both privacy and confidentiality, information collected about patients in the process of health-care delivery must be protected against unwarranted disclosure.

The importance of privacy and confidentiality has always been acknowledged. Medical privacy dates back over 2,000 years to the Hippocratic Oath, which compels physicians to keep confidential any information obtained during the attendance of the sick. Many other health-related professions have acknowledged the confidential nature of data obtained during the course of health-care delivery and have adopted similar oaths.

More recently, with an increase in automation, a number of governmental and nongovernmental entities have stressed the importance of confidentiality and security of health data. In 1994, the **Computer-Based Patient Record Institute** (CPRI) prepared a position paper on "Access to Patient Data." In the position paper, CPRI stressed that the establishment of a national regulatory framework to protect patients' informational privacy was of paramount importance to the success of the vision of the computer-based patient record. CPRI presented positions on four general areas concerned with access to patient data: (1) ownership of the primary patient record, (2) access of data by patients to their own health data, (3) access by others to patient-related data, and (4) levels of access. The nine specific positions held forth by CPRI are presented in Table 9-1.

Table 9-1. CPRI Position Statements on Access to Patient Data

1. Primary health records are the property of the health-care institution or licensed practitioner providing care; however, the information contained in the record belongs to the patient.

2. The right of privacy is a personal and fundamental right protected by the Constitution of the United States. Individuals have a right to privacy of their health information.

3. Health-care providers have an ethical and legal obligation to protect the confidentiality of all patient-identifiable information.

4. Only the patient or his/her legal representative has the right to authorize the disclosure of individually identifiable information to third parties.

5. Patients have the right to review the information contained in their health records.

6. Federal preemptive legislation should be enacted to address standard methodologies for the creation, authentication, retention, storage, access, disclosure, and admissibility of computer-based patient information. This legislation should also define and impose penalties for unauthorized use or disclosure of patient information.

7. Levels of access to computer-based patient records must be controlled through standardized computer security measures, business policies, procedures, access audit trails, penalties, and user education.

8. Standards governing access to patient data should be developed. These standards must include not only to whom and what level access may be granted, but also must define the purposes for which the information may be used.

9. Efforts must be made to educate consumers regarding computer-based patient records. Patients must have confidence in their right to access and control the release of their health information. Individuals must also have confidence in the ability of computer-based patient record systems to protect the security of their health information.

Numerous other governmental and nongovernmental groups have recognized the need to protect the privacy and confidentiality of health data and have released statements and/or positions regarding these issues. The American Health Information Management Association (AHIMA) has been a leading advocate for protecting the privacy and confidentiality of patient health data. Table 9-2 summarizes the publication of position statements by AHIMA. Among others who have also published reports, statements, or positions are the Institutes of Medicine (IOM), the Physician Payment Review Commission, the U.S. Department of Health and Human Services (DHHS), the General Accounting Office (GAO), the American Medical Association (AMA), and the American Hospital Association (AHA).

Legislative Protection of Privacy

The legislative protection of privacy of health data in the United States has historically been composed of a patchwork of privacy legislation on a state-by-state basis. There have been numerous attempts to enact national legislation that would prescribe a uniform federal health data privacy policy that would transcend state borders. The need for such a policy has become increasingly acknowledged as the country moves toward national health-care reform and as new technological applications, such as telemedicine, serve populations across state borders.

Table 9-2.   AHIMA Position Papers on Privacy and Confidentiality of Patient Data

Position Statements

- Patient Access to Personal Health Information
- Disclosure of Health Information
- Disclosure Relating to Alcohol and Drug Abuse Information
- Disclosure Relating to Adoption
- Redisclosure of Health Information
- Confidentiality of the Computer-Based Patient Record

One of the first efforts toward legislation of privacy was the enactment of the Federal Privacy Act of 1974. This act incorporated fair information practice principles outlined in a report prepared by the Advisory Committee on Automated Personal Data Systems under the auspices of the Department of Health, Education, and Welfare (HEW). The Privacy Act of 1974, however, covered data collection and maintenance by federal agencies and did not include data collected and maintained by the private sector. Thus, only hospitals operated by the federal government or private health-care or research institutions maintaining medical records under government contract are subject to the provisions of the act (Gostin et al., 1995).

An outgrowth of the Privacy Act was the establishment of the Privacy Protection Study Commission (PPSC). In 1977, this commission recommended the enactment of legislation that would include regulation of disclosures from patient medical records (Privacy Protection Study Commission, 1977). Several data protection measures were recommended that limited disclosures. These included prohibiting the use of information for reasons other than the purpose for which the disclosure was made; requiring individuals to be informed when disclosures were made without their specific authorization; and mandating the use of forms for authorization of disclosure. However, the enactment of legislation specific to the privacy of medical records was not accomplished. Various states and health organization accrediting bodies have adopted portions of the PPSC's recommendations. This piecemeal approach to the protection of informational privacy is not an adequate method and there "still remains the need for uniform interstate legislation" (Hallowell and Eldridge, 1988).

Another attempt at achievement of uniform national policy for health informational privacy was the adoption of the Uniform Health Care Information Act by the National Conference on Uniform State Laws in 1985. This attempt to establish uniformity and consistency in the protection of health information between the states has been unsuccessful as well. As of 1995, only Montana and Washington state had adopted the Uniform Health Care Information Act as state law.

Since 1993, with the advent of a movement toward health-care reform, several significant attempts have been made to enact federal legislation addressing the issues involving informational privacy. President Clinton's Health Security Act and other health-care reform bills introduced in Congress during 1994 all provided for the development of a health information infrastructure. A bill introduced by Representative Condit, called the

Fair Health Information Practices Act, provided for a comprehensive plan for the protection of health information. In May 1995, Senator Bond introduced the Health Information Modernization and Security Act. While this bill is aimed at improving the Medicare and Medicaid programs through the development of a health information network, it also specifically addresses issues related to data security and confidentiality. In October 1995, additional legislation was introduced by Senator Bennett titled the Medical Records Confidentiality Act of 1995. The purpose of this most recent legislative proposal is to establish uniform privacy protection for personally identifiable health information. The bill addresses the use and disclosure of all health treatment and payment information (not only Medicare and Medicaid data) throughout the United States. Specifically the Confidentiality Act includes the following (Frawley, 1995):

- Establishes uniform, comprehensive federal rules governing the use and disclosure of identifiable health information about individuals
- Specifies the responsibilities of those who collect, use, and maintain health information about individuals
- Provides mechanisms that will allow individuals to enforce their rights

This latest legislation was a combined effort among various organizations to develop drafting language for the bill. Among the participant groups were AHIMA, AHA, AMA, IBM, ACLU, and the Workgroup for Electronic Data Interchange (WEDI).

As the legislative history indicates, there has been an increasing awareness of the need to provide legislation at a national level addressing informational privacy issues. As of 1995, existing state laws are incomplete and inadequate to ensure informational privacy. The need for federal legislation is imperative if the United States hopes to build a national information infrastructure that supports health-care reform.

Security Fundamentals

Broadly speaking, any security program for health information should have three principal goals: (1) protecting the informational privacy of patient-related data, (2) ensuring the integrity of data, and (3) ensuring the availability of information to the appropriate individuals in a timely manner. The achievement of these goals can only be accomplished through the establishment of a sound information security organization and the implementation and coordination of multiple security strategies. Table 9-3 depicts the goals of an information security program and the informational security strategies that support each goal.

Later sections of this chapter discuss in detail each of the seven security strategies depicted in Table 9-3. However, it is important to recognize that no security program is complete unless all the security strategies are implemented to some extent. The degree of implementation of each strategy is dependent on the type and sensitivity of data that are collected, used, and maintained. It would be highly unusual to implement a health data security program without addressing all of the strategies outlined in Table 9-3.

Protecting Informational Privacy

There are many threats to informational privacy. The common methods used to compromise system security include (1) unauthorized user activity, (2) unauthorized access by either hackers or masqueraders, (3) unprotected downloaded files, and (4) use of Trojan horses.

Table 9-3.   Goals and Strategies of an Information Security Program

	Security Strategies						
Goals	**Security Organization**	**Risk Analysis**	**Business Continuity Planning**	**Data and Application Controls**	**Physical Controls**	**Access Controls**	**Network Security**
Informational Privacy	√	√		√	√	√	√
Information Integrity	√	√	√	√		√	√
Information Availability	√	√	√	√	√	√	√

Unauthorized User Activity

Unauthorized user activity occurs when authorized users of the system gain access to programs or files that they are not authorized to access. This is usually due to weak access controls, password sharing, or inefficient procedures to terminate system access by former employees. Instances of compromised information security are well documented in both popular and scholarly literature. In one instance, a disgruntled former employee planted a program that would wipe out all records of sales commissions. Even though the system break-in was discovered within 2 days, the company lost 168,000 records before disabling the program (Hafner et al., 1988). It is acknowledged that employees or former employees are the greatest risk in compromising data integrity (Gostin et al., 1995). In many of these instances, the compromise to data integrity is unintentional, for example, human error in data entry or the introduction of computer viruses. However, many times the corruption of data is intentional. Dowling (1980) cites several of these instances in hospital information systems.

Threats to data security are not limited to employees or former employees. There are many examples of "hackers" invading computer systems. A hacker is someone who bypasses the computer system's access controls by taking advantage of security weaknesses. Hackers frequently invade a computer system by gaining access to authorized user passwords. For example, in 1988, NASA's Jet Propulsion Laboratory in Pasadena, California, was invaded by hackers. In order to prevent future break-in attempts, NASA had spent 3 months changing passwords and clearing out trap-door programs that the intruders had planted to give them access (Hafner et al., 1988). Frequently, hacker access is accomplished through the use of multiple log-ons where the hacker tries different combinations of words sequentially in attempts to identify passwords. Hackers usually use computer programs, called demon programs, that are designed to sequentially search for valid passwords. A simple procedure that can discourage hacker password scanning is to limit the number of access attempts. For example, the user can be allowed 3 log-on attempts. Attempts to exceed the maximum number of log-ons can result in long delays that discourage hackers.

Downloaded Files

Another threat to confidentiality of data is the downloading of files from a secure environment to an unprotected environment. A common example is the downloading of files from a host computer to a microcomputer or local-area network so that data can be manipulated or processed locally. Such downloaded files could be easily copied to diskettes and surreptitiously distributed to unauthorized users or outsiders. Additionally such files may go unprotected in a local-area network environment where security measures are often weaker than in a mainframe environment.

Trojan Horses

The use of **Trojan horses** is another technique that is used to compromise informational privacy. A Trojan horse is a computer program used by hackers and other system intruders that masquerades as performing a useful or authorized function. The Trojan horse program also performs malicious functions unknown to the user. In the case of compromising confidential data, a Trojan horse may copy confidential files to unprotected areas of the system. Once resident on the user's system, the Trojan horse program can routinely copy confidential files to an area where the intruder has access. Many times, Trojan horse programs insert instructions into production computer programs. This method is frequently encountered when logic bombs or viruses are introduced to the production systems of computers.

Informational Privacy Models

There are several security models that are used to help ensure informational privacy. Each of these models uses various methods to classify data, users, and processes and implements techniques to limit access to data. One of the most common methods is the access control model (Tipton, 1993). The elements of this model were first presented in Chapter 6. Essentially this model (1) classifies data according to sensitivity, (2) classifies the subjects (users of data) who may read, write, or read and write data, and (3) authorizes the types of operations that may be performed on data. For example, a typical hierarchical data sensitivity classification used by the military is unclassified, confidential, secret, and top secret. IBM uses public, internal use only, confidential, confidential restricted, and registered confidential. In access control methods, users are customarily classified in groups according to organizational department or assigned projects. The final component of access control is the identification of the kinds of operations that a subject (user) can perform on the data. For example, this would include no privileges at all, read, write and read, and write only privileges and specifying the data on which the user can perform these functions. Specifics regarding access control methods are presented later in this chapter.

Protecting Data Integrity

In the context of data security, data integrity means the protection of data and programs from accidental or unauthorized intentional change. A data security program cannot ensure the accuracy of data. However, it should be able to ensure that data entered into the system are protected from unauthorized modification or deletion and that accidental changes are minimized. In the clinical environment, it is obvious why the integrity of data must be protected. Quality patient care and, in fact, the lives of patients rely on data being reliable. Mistakes in medication orders or dosages, ordering of diagnostic or therapeutic procedures, or incorrect patient-care documentation could adversely impact the quality of patient care. In addition to clinical data, errors in financial records could adversely impact facility reimbursement or result in loss of enterprise assets.

Maintaining the integrity of data, just like maintaining the confidentiality of data, relies on good access control. Like informational privacy, the integrity of data can be compromised by hackers, unauthorized users, unprotected downloaded files, and Trojan horses. In addition, however, authorized users can corrupt data through data entry errors or mistakes in modifications and deletions of data.

Data Integrity Protection Models

As discussed in Chapter 6, there are several ways in which the integrity of data can be protected: (1) preventing unauthorized users from making data modifications; (2) preventing authorized users from making unauthorized modifications; (3) preventing authorized users from making errors; and (4) establishing procedures and using techniques to maintain internal consistency of data. Data integrity is not only concerned with preserving the integrity of the data elements themselves. Another important part of the integrity model is to ensure that the system performs the way it was intended—consistently and reliably. There are a variety of different models that help to ensure data integrity, for example, Biba, Goguen-Meseguer,

Sutherland, Clark-Wilson and Brewer-Nash. The details of some of these models are presented later in this chapter.

Ensuring Data Availability

A security program must ensure the availability of data to end-users—that is, the system should provide the appropriate data to the appropriate user at the appropriate time. Unavailability of data can result from either denial of service or from loss of data processing functions due to natural disasters such as fires, storms, or from human actions such as malicious attacks.

Denial of service usually results because of system intrusion, for example, the introduction of a **worm** into a computer network system. A worm is a program that reproduces by copying itself from one system to another while traveling from machine to machine over a computer network. The result of a worm attack is usually degradation of the system, making normal functioning unavailable to users.

The loss of computing services is more often due to human error or to natural disaster. For example, in one hospital computer data center a major ancillary computer system (laboratory) was taken down due to housekeeping personnel inadvertently unplugging the host computer. Natural disasters such as fires, storms, tornadoes, and earthquakes can result in major destruction of a data center or interruption of service. Because of the potential for significant loss, it is essential that each information service develop a contingency plan. This plan is often called a business continuity plan, whose purpose is to provide an alternate means of processing data when natural or human disasters strike. The plan usually provides for alternative site processing and for recovery of data following disasters. The components of a business continuity plan are addressed in more detail in later sections of this chapter.

Conclusion

There are three primary purposes of a data security program: protecting informational privacy, ensuring data integrity, and providing availability of data to end-users. The emphasis on these goals varies by industry. For example, informational privacy may be less of an issue in systems that maintain inventory control. In the health-care industry, all three facets of a security program are equally important. If any one of the three components of a data security program are weak in a health-care enterprise, the organization opens itself to numerous problems. If a patient's confidentiality is breached, there may be legal ramifications. If data integrity is not maintained, patient care may be adversely impacted or financial loss may occur. Likewise, the unavailability of data can contribute to suboptimal patient care or result in financial loss. The need to provide a security program that addresses all three issues—informational privacy, data integrity, and data availability—is a primary reason why health data security programs can be very complex to develop as well as to maintain.

Establishing a Security Program

The need for data security programs and development of organizational structures to support such programs is being recognized by health-care enterprises today. This recognition is the result of the industry's continued growing dependence on information technology, that information is an organizational asset, and that expanded connectivity is occurring internal and external to the enterprise. In the 1980s, data security principally involved protection of confidential patient information usually found in paper records. Issues involving data integrity and data availability were less emphasized because most of the operational activity of a health-care facility was not computerized. This situation has changed dramatically and all aspects of data security have become a priority for health-care enterprises.

Today, it is not unusual to find acute-care facilities, health maintenance organizations, clinics, and other health-care facilities highly dependent on automation. For the most part, automated financial information systems, which include accounting and financial management systems, are prevalent. Basic core functions such as registration, admission, discharge, and transfer (RADT) systems are automated in acute-care facilities. Ancillary departments such as laboratory, pharmacy, and radiology are frequently automated and interfaced or integrated into the RADT core systems. Additionally, patient-care-related activities such as medication administration and nursing-care documentation are more and more frequently automated. In the outpatient setting, there has been enormous activity in computerizing the patient record. While these efforts do not necessarily incorporate the fundamental elements of a **computer-based patient record** (CPR) as delineated by the Institutes of Medicine (IOM), they nonetheless are evidence of increasing dependence on automated information systems.

There is a growing recognition in the health-care arena that information is an organizational asset. The security, integrity, and availability of data are critical for the success of an enterprise. It is important from both patient and organizational perspectives that informational privacy is maintained. Because of the competitive nature of health care today, it is critical for organizations to ensure that data are private.

The interconnectivity among health-care enterprises has spurred the need for more sophisticated security programs. The introduction of local-area and wide-area networks opens up an entire new frontier of security problems. The development of integrated delivery systems (IDS) and dependence on **electronic data interchange** (EDI), which rely on the use of various networks and interconnections among computer systems, offer a host of problems involving not only informational privacy, but data integrity and availability as well. The use of the Internet as a tool for information seeking and gathering has also played an important role in recognizing the need for more sophisticated security programs. However, probably one of the principal elements in heightening security program awareness is the discussion of plans for the development of a national health-care information infrastructure (NII). Security, perhaps, is the single most important policy issue facing the development of automated health information systems. As Gostin and colleagues (1995) note, "the success of the health care system depends in large part on the integrity of information and the confidence of the public that private information will be vigorously protected."

Although information security awareness has been heightened during the past few years, historically hospitals have not had broad security programs. In a recent survey, results indicated that hospitals should be doing more to protect sensitive data (Gordon, Fogel, and McKenzie, 1993). The survey revealed that hospitals with over 800 beds and urban hospitals had greater controls in place to protect patient information than smaller hospitals. For example, 88 percent of hospitals with over 800 beds indicated they had a written policy on the use of patient records while only 63 percent of hospitals with fewer than 400 beds indicated they had such a written policy. The survey also showed that, on a whole, hospitals were taking too long to terminate system access of former employees. Only 54 percent of all hospitals surveyed required that all employees sign confidentiality agreements and only 33 percent required consultants to sign confidentiality agreements. The results also showed that while hospitals maintained basic security restrictions on access to patient databases, they did not have similar policies or restrictions in place on the printing of patient data nor could most track who was accessing sensitive patient data. The results of such surveys indicate the urgent need for the development of enterprise-wide security programs in health-care organizations.

Components of a Security Program

Data security programs should be concerned not only with technological issues and methods but should also address human resource issues. To be successful the design of a security program must address the needs of the organization. A balance must be struck between the amount of security necessary and the cost/benefit of the program to the organization. For example, biometric authentication procedures such as retinal scans or fingerprints may be justified in a high-security military environment but may be cost prohibitive and/or unnecessary for the protection of data in a health-care clinic or physician's office. The first principle, therefore, in establishing a security program is that the security organizational structure, technological controls, and policies and procedures implemented must meet the requirements of the organization.

Determining the Scope of the Security Program

A successful security program must be broad enough to include all automated information systems in the organization. Frequently in health-care facilities the information systems department will have good security measures in place for the mainframe system. However, security measures are deficient for ancillary systems, networks, and personal computers throughout the organization.

An inventory of information systems throughout the enterprise should be undertaken. The inventory should include identification of hardware, software applications, and networks within the organization as an initial analysis for identification of security program scope. Once the inventory is completed, a risk assessment should be performed. The techniques of risk assessment are described in a later section of this chapter. Briefly, however, the risk assessment includes identifying the role played by each of the information systems in the enterprise, how vital the role is in the overall functioning of the organization, and the adverse impact on the organization if security is breached. The results of the risk assessment will provide the foundation for identifying and evaluating safeguards and for a cost-benefit analysis. There are a variety of software tools that can assist in the risk analysis. Both quantitative and qualitative measures are usually used in conducting the risk assessment.

Security Program Organization

It is not unusual to find that there is no formal data security organizational structure in health-care facilities. Frequently data security is limited to automated systems under the direct control of the information systems department and there is no formal structure that addresses informational privacy, integrity, or business continuity planning on an enterprise-wide basis. The weakness with this type of approach is obvious. Ancillary systems such as laboratory, radiology, human resource management, and decision support are just as critical to an organization as core systems run on mainframe computers. If data are corrupted or destroyed in nonprotected systems, this situation might have a serious a consequence as the loss or destruction of data on mainframe systems. Thus, an appropriate security organizational structure must be developed that has oversight and responsibility for informational privacy, data integrity, and data availability on an enterprise-wide basis. The positioning of the security structure will depend on the organization. The information security structure can be housed in the information systems department, the corporate security department if the health-care facility has one, the risk management department, or the internal audit department. In some organizations the position of **chief security officer** (CSO) has been created. The CSO may report directly to the chief executive officer (CEO), indicating that the position carries enterprise-wide responsibility for data security management. Typical functions of a CSO are included in Table 9-4.

A security program, because of its multifaceted purposes, is multidisciplinary—no one person will likely have the knowledge and skills to staff the security function. In order to provide the appropriate mix of skills to carry out the security function, a matrix organizational structure might be considered. This would include representatives from internal auditing and

Table 9-4.   Typical Functions of a Chief Security Officer

- Participate in facility strategic planning process, identifying security needs of new systems development.
- In concert with the hospital data security committee, develop hospital-wide information security policy.
- Develop security procedures and standards in accordance with the hospital data security policy.
- Administer and coordinate the administration of security software for the hospital mainframes, minicomputers, and personal computers. This includes establishing security controls and extracting and evaluating audit information.
- Manage hospital confidentiality agreements. This includes ensuring that hospital confidentiality agreements are signed by all staff and investigating and reporting violations of the hospital data security policy.
- Coordinate data security activities of all hospital local-area network administrators. This includes ensuring that LAN security procedures are up to date and that regular server backups are made and stored in a safe place away from the location of the server.
- Provide user training on security issues.
- Monitor audit trail records to identify security violations.
- Develop and monitor procedures for timely updating and/or removal of access rights of individuals who transfer within the organization or those who resign or are terminated from the organization.
- Provide internal consulting assistance on implementing security controls.
- Conduct risk assessment of facility information systems.

information systems auditing, legal and risk management departments, quality assurance, data administration, and computer operations and technical support. Whatever the skill and person mix, the security organization must be thoroughly knowledgeable about the threats and vulnerabilities faced by a health-care organization.

Because an enterprise-wide security function is a relatively new concept to health-care organizations, little data are available on full-time-equivalent (FTE) employee ratios relative to other facility functions. However, in other industries surveys have shown that the ratio of FTEs in information security to those in information systems is 1 percent to 5 percent, the average being slightly less than 3 percent (Wood, 1993).

The security organization should include the formation of a security policy advisory committee. Major departments of the facility should be represented on the advisory committee to voice the organization's various business interests and technological environments. The purpose of the committee is to assist the chief security officer (CSO) in the development of enterprise-wide security policy. The benefit of such a group is that buy-in from user groups is readily obtained in support of procedures and policies established. The advisory committee should be established by the executive management of the organization and given a clear charge of its duties and responsibilities. Such high management support indicates to the rest of the organization the importance that is being placed on security management within the enterprise. Normally the CSO will chair the advisory group.

Security Policies, Procedures, and Standards

The implementation, monitoring, and follow-up measures of a security program are heavily people dependent. In conjunction with the facility security policy advisory committee, the CSO should be responsible for the development of enterprise-wide security policies and standards. Individual procedures that support policy should be reviewed by the CSO and advisory committee to ensure that they support the enterprise security policies.

Typically, an organizational security policy manual is developed. This manual includes an overriding enterprise security directive that emphasizes the importance of information as an asset to the organization and holds all employees responsible for its protection. The policy manual will also delineate the responsibilities of management, security staff, and employees in protection of the information asset.

Standards relating to information classification should also be specified in the policy manual. This includes what standard will be used in classifying information into (1) availability categories (i.e., vital, important, useful, nonessential), (2) integrity categories (i.e., critical, sensitive, valuable, noncritical), and (3) confidentiality categories (i.e., registered confidential, confidential, internal use only, public). Security standards for all automated information systems, systems development, data processing operations, and personnel administration should be included in the enterprise-wide security manual.

Conclusion

The importance of establishing an enterprise-wide security program in health-care organizations is well recognized. Such a program must have top management support and direction if it is to be successful. The program must be supported by sufficient resources to accomplish its goals of protecting informational privacy and integrity and ensuring data availability. The scope of the security program must be sufficiently broad to encompass all vital organizational information systems and resources. An appropriate organizational structure must be established to ensure that adequate polices and procedures are developed, implemented, and monitored. As health care moves toward more automation and integration of internal and external data sources, the importance of informational security programs as an integral part of the organizational structure will continue to be recognized.

Risk Analysis and Management

An important part of any security program is the management of risk. Risk management deals with the identification, management, and control of untoward events. Automated systems are subject to many types of risks that may corrupt data, or interfere with or shut down computer operations. Some of these risks include human error, internal and external sabotage, technological defects, and natural disasters. The dilemma for any organization in addressing these threats is determining the appropriate level and kind of security controls that should be implemented. In today's cost-conscious environment implementation of security controls must be cost justified and a balance must be achieved between benefit and cost.

Two very important security processes are based on the data gathered from the **risk analysis** and **assessment:** (1) identification and development of countermeasures to protect the information resources and (2) development of a business continuity plan (frequently called the disaster plan). The development of countermeasures and the business continuity plan are at the heart of the security program. There is a correlation between a good risk assessment and the implementation of appropriate security controls. When a risk assessment has not been performed or has been poorly done, it is highly likely that the security program is extremely weak and vulner-

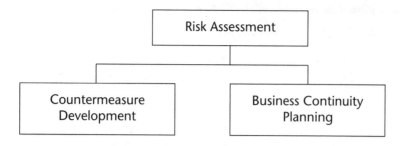

Figure 9-1.   Relationship between Risk Assessment and Countermeasure and Business Continuity Planning

able both to unintentional and intentional threats. Figure 9-1 shows the relationship between the risk assessment process and countermeasure development and business continuity planning.

The following sections describe the details of conducting a risk assessment. Remember that the results of the analysis and subsequent assessment are critical elements to both the development of appropriate countermeasures to prevent and control risk and for the development of the organizational business continuity plan.

Risk Analysis

Conducting a risk analysis is an essential first component of managing security threats. Risk analysis entails (1) the identification of threats or risks to security, (2) the measurement of how likely it is that these risks will occur, and (3) the estimation of impact if the harmful event were to occur. Risks to security include data entry error, unauthorized physical access to data, internal and external sabotage, power failure or fluctuation, and malfunction or failure of the central processing unit. Table 9-5 presents a list of potential threats and risks.

While we can make a list of adverse events, the list is relatively useless unless we know what the expected occurrence of the risks are. For instance, how many times per day can we expect data entry error to occur? How often will a power failure happen? How many times can we expect that data will be corrupted by external sabotage of the system? Estimation

Table 9-5. Potential Threats and Risks

Unintentional Threats	Natural Disasters	Internal flood
		External flood
		Internal fire
		External fire
		Tornado
		Earthquake
		Snowstorm
	Equipment Failure	Power failure
		System software failure
		Application software failure
		Hardware failure
		Network failure
	Human Error	Data entry error
		Coffee/drink spill
		Unplugging of equipment
		Improper handling of sensitive data
Intentional Threats	Theft	Personal computers
		Components
		Printers
		Software
		Data
		Unauthorized access to data or programs
	Fraud	Unauthorized modification of software
		Unauthorized access to data
	Malice	Damage of software
		Damage of data

of the occurrence of such risks is important if efficient and cost-effective countermeasures are to be put in place.

Identification of Assets

The first step in conducting a risk analysis is to know what constitutes the organizational information assets. The scope of identifying the assets depends on whether or not an enterprise-wide analysis is being conducted or if the analysis is application specific. For most purposes, it is sufficient to broadly identify assets. For example, in an integrated delivery system (IDS) that includes a hospital and clinic, the assets may be broadly defined as shown in Table 9-6. The identification of information assets can be done through interviews with users, departments (i.e., owners of information and systems), and managers. Additionally information can be gathered from existing information systems inventories and/or the organizational accounting office.

Evaluating Information Assets

Once the informational assets have been identified, they should to be evaluated in terms of their value to the organization. For example, how necessary is each of the applications in Table 9-6 to the continuity of the organization's critical operations? Criticality is based on several factors. Among these are legal and regulatory requirements, loss of revenue, type of service loss (i.e., patient care, administrative, financial), and image impact on the organization. To help quantify the value of an informational asset, a scale can be developed. Table 9-7 includes the information assets for one IDS and how that organization ranked the system criticality. It is important to recognize that not all similar systems will be ranked with the same criticality. The criticalness of the system will be specific to the organization.

While the criticalness of a system may be categorized as a scale as we saw in Table 9-7, frequently criticality is defined as the **annualized loss expectancy** (ALE). ALE is usually defined as the financial impact or loss to the organization should the system fail. ALE is typically calculated by determining what the financial loss would be for each occurrence of a

Table 9-6. Sample Assets of an Integrated Delivery System

Order Entry/Results Reporting

Payroll

Laboratory

Pharmacy

Critical-Care Monitoring/Documentation

Patient Admitting/Discharge

Radiology

Table 9-7.　Information Assets and Criticality Score

Information Asset	Criticality Level
Order Entry/Results Reporting	1
Payroll	1
Laboratory	1
Pharmacy	1
Critical-Care Monitoring/Documentation	1
Patient Admitting/Discharge	1
Radiology	3

1 = Extremely high, 2 = very high, 3 = medium, 4 = low, 5 = very low.

harmful event multiplied by the number of times the event is expected to happen within 1 year. Say that an organization knows that a significant power failure has a probability of occurring once per year. Also assume that the organization knows the type and amount of cost associated with a power outage that caused all critical systems to go down for a certain period of time. These costs, for instance, might include additional staffing to run manual backups of critical systems, outsourcing costs for procedures needing to be performed during system failure, estimated lost revenue, and extension of billing recovery time. Having this information, the organization can then calculate how much the ALE would be for a major power failure that would occur once per year. Table 9-8 depicts a hypothetical situation where major power failure with a probability of happening once per year results in a 1-day outage of critical systems.

An essential element of calculating the ALE as depicted in Table 9-8 is knowing the probability of a harmful event and the costs associated with the event. These data may be obtained from historical organizational information. For instance, how many times has a certain event occurred in the past and what was the resultant loss? Consulting companies and other security references also produce disaster probability occurrence tables.

Frequently hard cost data are not available to the organization to determine the ALE. In these cases, a more qualitative approach is taken. Rather than including dollar amounts in the formula, risk is calculated as some function of the probability of occurrence of a harmful event equal to some function of the level of threat and the level of vulnerability (Buck, 1991).

Table 9-8. Annualized Loss Expectancy for Critical Systems: One-Time Power Failure for 1 Day Downtime

Information System	Additional Personnel Cost	Other Expenses
Order Entry/Results Reporting	$25,000 in additional clerical staff/overtime	
Laboratory System	$5,000 in additional staff/overtime	$25,000 in outsourcing procedures; estimate 10% lost revenue per day
Radiology	$2,000 in additional staff/overtime	Estimate 10% lost revenue per day
Pharmacy	$3,000 in additional staff/overtime	10% lost charge volumes

Risk Analysis Methods

The student should be aware that there are many methodologies for determining risk. Even though methodologies differ significantly in complexity levels of calculation/computation, they all try to divide the problem of risk into measurable parts. Usually these methodologies also make a distinction between the calculation of risk based on unintentional and intentional occurrences. For example, calculation of risk based on unintentional occurrences (i.e., power failures, data entry errors), are usually based on the probability of the occurrence of the event and its cost impact. This method was demonstrated in Table 9-8. However, there are different formulae used for the calculation of intentional threats such as fraud, malice, and sabotage, because the risk of an intentional threat is based on such factors as the attractiveness of a system to a specific perpetrator, the availability of the system to perpetrator attack, and the vulnerability of the system. An example of such a formula is the Stanford Institute's Relative Impact Measure (Nelson, 1978). This formula categorizes the types of perpetrator classes, the severity rating for the perpetrator class, the probability of vulnerability linking the perpetrator class with the target system, the relative attractiveness of the target class to the perpetrators, and the impact of the success of an attack on the target system. Table 9-9 lists the differences in factors used to calculate unintentional and intentional harmful occurrences.

Table 9-9.   Factors Influencing Determination of Risk for Unintentional and Intentional Harmful Occurrences

Unintentional Occurrences	Intentional Occurrences
• Probability of occurrence	• Number of individuals in perpetrator class
• Estimated loss	• Severity rating for perpetrator class
	• Vulnerability of the system to a specific perpetrator class
	• Attractiveness of the system to a specific class of perpetrator
	• Impact of success of harmful occurrence

The calculation of risk, no matter what formulae are used, usually has a subjective component. Risk assessment is a "soft" science and the ultimate determination of risk is based on management judgment. How specific can the probability be determined that links a specific perpetrator class to a target system? How more probable is it that programmers are more likely perpetrators of a system than clerical personnel or outside hackers in a hospital system? The probability estimates, if not based on historical statistical data, are likely to be arbitrary measurements based on judgment and experience of the organizational security team.

Sample Risk Assessment

Once the data have been collected in the risk analysis, a detailed risk assessment must be performed. To demonstrate the product of a risk assessment, the following hypothetical scenario is used:

TGL is an integrated delivery system consisting of four hospitals, four clinics, a skilled nursing facility, and home health agency. TGL wants to conduct a risk assessment of its information systems. Initially the assessment will include only the largest acute-care facility in the system and the largest clinic.

Step 1: Identification of the Information Assets

The scope of the risk assessment is system-wide as opposed to application specific. The risk assessment team has determined that the assessment should be broad in scope and focus will be information system specific, as opposed to doing a risk assessment based on hardware and software inventories. The TGL has identified the information systems depicted in Table 9-10 as critical to the operation of both the hospital and clinic.

Step 2: Identification of the Criticality of Information Systems

Once the informational system assets were identified, TGL determined the criticality of each system to the overall operation of the selected hospital and clinic. The criticality scale was an arbitrary measure based on the best judgment of the security team and user department interviews. Considerations in assigning a criticality level to the system included overall operational impact, patient-care impact, financial impact, and legal issues. Table 9-11 depicts the criticality level assigned to each major system.

Step 3: Risk Analysis

Once the criticality of the systems had been determined, the security team identified the potential threats that could occur to the system. The team chose to calculate a risk measurement index rather than using the ALE

Table 9-10.   Critical Information Systems for TGL Integrated Delivery System

Order Entry/Results Reporting
Payroll
Laboratory
Pharmacy
Critical-Care Monitoring/Documentation
Patient Admitting/Discharge
Radiology
Clinic Scheduling
Accounts Payable
Accounts Receivable
Materials Management

Table 9-11. Criticality Level for each TGL System

Information Asset	Criticality Level
Order Entry/Results Reporting	1
Payroll	1
Laboratory	1
Pharmacy	1
Critical-Care Monitoring/Documentation	1
Patient Admitting/Discharge	1
Radiology	3
Clinic Scheduling	3
Accounts Payable	2
Accounts Receivable	2
Materials Management	4

1 = extremely high, 2 = very high, 3 = medium, 4 = low, 5 = very low.

method for risk assessment. They decided to do this because the ALE only provides one measurement of impact—financial impact—and does not take into consideration other operational elements such as patient care, administrative, or legal impacts.

To perform this type of risk measurement index and evaluation, the event probability was identified as well as the vulnerability level of each system. Given these data, the security team then determined an overall risk factor for each potential threat. An arbitrary scale of 1 to 3 was used to indicate whether the risks were high, medium, or low. A sample of the evaluation for the order-entry/results reporting system is provided in Table 9-12. For each of the critical systems, the security team performed a similar analysis. The results of the analysis for all systems then provided the foundation for the determination of countermeasures that should be in place to protect the various systems.

Development of Countermeasures

Once the risk assessment is completed and the risk level associated with each threat for every system is identified, then the security team must determine appropriate countermeasures. A balance must be struck between the cost of the countermeasure and the level of protection that is required for each system. In the case of TGL, the team took into account

Table 9-12. Risk Assessment Order-Entry/Results Reporting System: Unintentional Event

Order-Entry/Results Reporting System			*System Criticality Level: 1*		
Threat	*System Vulnerability Level*	*Event Probability*	*Operational Impact*	*Financial Impact*	*Risk Level*
Internal fire	3	3	1	1	3
Internal flood	3	3	1	1	3
Power failure	1	1	1	2	2
CPU failure	1	2	1	2	2
System software failure	1	1	1	2	1
Application software failure	1	1	1	2	1
Data entry error	1	1	1	2	1

1 = high, 2 = medium, 3 = low.

the criticality level of each system and the risk level score. For those events with a high level risk score associated with a highly critical system, the team chose to implement higher sophisticated countermeasures. The types of countermeasures varied based on the type of risk or threat. Various countermeasures are discussed in detail in the next section of this chapter.

Prevention and Control Countermeasures

The objective of countermeasures is to either (1) prevent a harmful event from occurring or (2) control the damage of the event after it has occurred by minimizing the impact of the event and maximizing the recovery. Countermeasures may be grouped into the following categories:

- Personnel security
- Physical security
- Hardware security
- Software security
- Communications security

Each of these categories is discussed in detail in the following sections.

Personnel Security

Because one of the greatest threats to security is the organization's employees, good personnel security measures must be implemented. To implement a successful personnel security program, there must be top management commitment. Executive-level management must support the concept of security and set a vision for employees. This vision can be communicated through employee publications, orientation, and regularly scheduled management and employee meetings. To support commitment to security, top management must (1) endorse security policies and procedures, (2) provide the resources to implement these policies and procedures, and (3) provide a security structure that has oversight over the entire security program. Where a chief security officer is appointed, visibility to the importance of the security initiative is highlighted, particularly if this individual sits on the executive team and reports directly to the CEO.

Security Procedures in Employee Hiring

Good personnel security begins at the time of hiring employees. All job position descriptions should include the level of information access (security clearance) for each employee. Employees should only have access to information on a need-to-know basis. Although the security access level is usually assigned by employee job title and/or group membership by the information systems department, it is equally important for the employee to know his or her security level at the time of employment.

All employees should be provided with orientation training to the organization's security and privacy policies. The extent of the orientation will be dependent on the employee's organizational level and level of access to information. Orientation training should minimally include review of the organization's security policies and procedures, appropriate to job classification; delineation of employee responsibilities; and review of procedures for reporting security and privacy violations.

The organization should have a professional code of ethics in regard to information security. This code should be given to the employee at the time of hiring. The expectation that every employee is bound by this code should be enforced through a written, signed, and dated pledge of confidentiality or confidentiality agreement. The confidentiality agreement should state that the employee has been made aware of the health organization's security and privacy policy and understands the consequences of breaching the policy. The signed confidentiality agreement should become part of the employee's personnel file. Unfortunately, studies have shown that only about 50 percent of hospitals require employees to sign such confidentiality agreements (Gordon, Fogel, and McKenzie, 1993).

In addition to orientation training in security and privacy, the organization should provide regular, periodic training sessions for all employees. This may be done on an annual basis and a certificate of attendance at such workshops could be put in the employee's personnel file. For jobs entailing the handling of large amounts of sensitive data and/or access to computer hardware and software, a thorough evaluation of the prospective employee's background should be conducted, including reference checks from previous employers.

Change in Job Function or Termination

Certain security procedures should be in place whenever an employee changes a job within the organization or leaves or is terminated from the organization. When an employee changes jobs within the organization, the information systems department should be immediately contacted so that security access clearance can be changed. Old clearances should be deleted immediately at the time of job change and should not be postponed for days or weeks. Depending on the job classification, clearance may be lowered or highered. Whatever the case, employees should be notified of their different access rights and their responsibilities.

In cases where the employee leaves the organization or is terminated, information access privileges must be revoked immediately. This means that all user IDs and passwords be revoked; that control items (such as keys or badges) be retrieved; and that all hardware, software, or documentation issued to the employee be retrieved. Unfortunately, studies have indicated that hospitals are taking too long to revoke former employee privileges. In one study, almost half of the respondents said that it took longer than a day to cancel a user's access to the system (Gordon, Fogel, and McKenzie, 1993). This situation is intolerable in any organization, particularly in light of studies that have indicated that former disgruntled employees are a major threat to security.

Corrective and Disciplinary Action

As previously discussed, security policies and procedures need to delineate the consequences of employee breach of security. Consequences may be include immediate termination of an employee, suspension without pay for a stipulated period, or written or verbal warnings. The severity of the consequence should be based on the level of the breach. Unintentional acts, such as data entry or other human error, may require verbal or written warnings regarding performance. Intentional acts, such as invasion of patient privacy, theft, fraud, or malice, require harsher consequences such as job suspension or termination.

The process by which intentional breeches of security are investigated should be documented in the organization's security policies and procedures. An intentional breach may be identified through regular reviews of computer audit trails, identification of corrupted data files or programs, or from witnesses' reports. Once a breach has been identified, it should be systematically investigated. This may mean gathering additional evidence from witnesses, from computer-generated materials such as audit trails, from existing documents and reports, or from a video tape security system. In some organizations, determination of the occurrence of an intentional breach is made by a security committee. In other cases, the determination may be made by the chief security officer. Whatever the process, once the bulk of the evidence indicates a breach of security, institutional personnel and security policies should be followed to determine and implement consequences.

Physical Security

Physical protection of the information resource encompasses many components including (1) data resources are housed in well-constructed buildings safe from natural and intentional security threats and (2) fire and other safety codes are in compliance with local ordinances. In addition, physical security includes implementing the appropriate level of preventive controls, such as ensuring that access to computer hardware, software, and data storage is limited to authorized personnel.

Physical Location

Physical security begins with the selection of the site for the data center. The data center is the hub for all information processing of the organization. It includes computers, data storage, and communications that usually link the entire enterprise. Even though data processing may be distributed (i.e., performed on multiple mainframes, mini- and microcomputers and servers), the physical location of much of the equipment will be in the data center. Thus, the data center must be located in a building where the threat of fire, water damage, corrosive agents, and smoke is limited. Areas adjacent to the data center should be investigated to determine if there are any potential hazards. For example, data centers should not be located near areas where there may be electromagnetic radiation. The organization should ensure that the data center meets all fire, building, and electrical codes to minimize unintentional threats.

Physical Access

Only authorized personnel should have access to the data center. The data center should not be accessible from the street or ground level. The number of areas housing computer hardware, software, and data should be kept to a minimum and secured by using keypads, card readers, or card swipe mechanisms. Personnel should be required at all times to wear an organizational identification badge. Minimally such a badge should contain the name, photograph, and signature of the badge holder, organizational job and department titles, badge serial number and expiration date. Such badges can also be designed with magnetic strips to function in card readers or swipe mechanisms.

For visitors, vendors, and other organizational personnel who occasionally need access to the data center, there should be a reception area. An access control log should be maintained and should record the following information: identification of visitor; employer or affiliation; purpose of visit; date and time of entry; date and time of departure; and name of authorized employee who is requesting entry and who will accompany the visitor through the data center. Visitors to the data center should be identified with a visitor's badge.

Fire, Utilities, and other Protections

Rarely do fires occur in computers themselves since their material components are intrinsically noncombustible. When fires do occur within the equipment itself, it is usually due to the malfunction of some component part. In these cases, the fire can usually be easily detected and eliminated with a fire extinguisher.

The major source of fires in a data computer center is from electrical distribution systems. There are many causes of these kinds of fires including improper installation of electrical equipment and overloaded circuits. Therefore, to prevent these types of fires, the security program should have standard operating procedures for the installation, monitoring, and maintenance of all electrical equipment and wiring for computers, support equipment, and environmental equipment such as air conditioners.

To prevent and control fires, fire detection systems should be in place. The most efficient detection system is a smoke-detection system that can sense smoke before flames erupt. The detection system should sound both a local alarm and one to a centralized security monitoring area. Suppression of fires can be accomplished by water sprinkler systems, gaseous flooding systems, and fire extinguishers. There has been considerable debate over the use of water sprinklers or gaseous flooding systems that use substances such as Halon. There has been recent concern about the use of Halon because of environmental damage caused by chlorofluorocarbons, and use of Halon will likely be prohibited in the near future. Fire extinguishers should be of a mix of water, carbon dioxide, and Halon 1211. All staff should be trained in fire extinguisher use.

The data center needs to be protected from electrical outages and malfunctions. The voltage to the data center must to be sufficiently regulated to prevent power surges, voltage reductions, and other disturbances. In cases where there is a complete electrical outage, an uninterruptable power supply (UPS) service is essential. A UPS service provides electrical power for a specified period of time, allowing systems to either run uninterrupted or to be gradually brought down by information systems personnel so that minimum damage and data loss are incurred.

Damage to the data center by water is another security threat. Water detection equipment should be installed and there should be a plan for adequate drainage of water.

Hardware Security

All hardware should be installed and maintained according to manufacturer instructions. Policies and procedures should be in place for periodic hardware maintenance. Inventories must be available for all hardware devices along with a log of scheduled and unscheduled maintenance checks or procedures for each device. A contact log of vendors, support personnel, and field service personnel should be maintained as well for each hardware device. Employees responsible for maintenance should be knowledgeable and should attend training sessions to update skills.

In addition to installation and maintenance procedures, hardware security features should be used to prevent and minimize risk, including automatic power-down capabilities in instances where environmental conditions become a potential risk; and over-temperature, over-humidity, and under-voltage detection. The system should also be capable of producing hardware error control logs. These logs should contain records of instruction or command retries, data transfer retries, and error conditions.

Systems should be able to identify authorized terminals, workstations, or personal computers. The system should be able to identify each user or unit by hardware means, use encryption methods, and use dedicated communications.

Software Security

Like hardware security, the mechanisms to protect software include good practices in the development and purchase of software, quality assurance and testing of software, security features, and elements of database management.

Software Development Life Cycle

Establishing procedures for software development is critical to ensuring proper functioning of information systems. The systems development life cycle (SDLC) contains steps for the identification of data flow, system function, programming, database development, prototype development, testing, and implementation. It is essential that security concerns are addressed up front in any development effort. The information systems function must have procedures in place in the SDLC including security concerns. When software, databases, or prototype systems are developed, they should go through systematic testing prior to implementation.

Systematic testing of newly developed or changed software requires that test criteria be established—that is, what functions must the system adequately perform. Input from users should be obtained in developing the test criteria in order to ensure that both content and function are present in the system. For example, in an order entry system, we would expect that the system would correctly process an order for a laboratory test. Criteria relating to the correct processing of the order would be established. This might mean that the correct patient identification was transmitted from the RADT system; that a complete array of tests could be chosen by the physician from a menu on the terminal; that the test could be ordered 1, 2, or 3 days in advance; that the date and time when the test was ordered were documented; and so on.

It is important to separate the new software from the production environment, because the production environment should not be subjected to any potential software or programming errors that might affect its operation. Therefore, once test criteria are established, test data should be created. These test data should then be run through the system to determine whether or not the system functions as planned. Results of system testing and user acceptance testing should be reviewed to ensure that the system operates as intended.

To ensure that software is functioning appropriately, a change management process must be made part of an information systems function. In this case, change management means managing changes made in software, programs, and databases. The change management process outlines how requests for software changes are made and provides mechanisms for the tracking and recording of changes. The change management program documents what changes were made to the affected software, how these changes were made, who made the changes, when the changes became operational, and when the changes were tested. A change management log is maintained of all changes made to software, programs, or databases.

Purchase of Software

Software purchased from an outside vendor requires testing as well as software and applications developed in-house. Security procedures should be in place for examining purchased software for viruses, logic bombs, or other destructive functions. Such destructive functions can spread rapidly within an organization, causing havoc to regular operations.

Control of Software

An inventory of software and databases must be maintained, including all applications; all programs; databases and files; command and script files; software utilities; systems software; warranty/maintenance conditions; and vendor contact name, address, and phone number. The inventory should include the number of copies of each piece of software and its location(s). The owner and/or custodian of each piece of software should also be identified in the inventory. The date the software was created and its version/level number should be included. Dates of modifications and who was authorized to make changes should be entered in the inventory. The inventory should contain configuration charts for software, databases, and communication components. The charts should define interdependencies among applications. A copy of the inventory should be maintained off-site for disaster recovery purposes.

In addition to the inventory, there should be standard operating policies and procedures for the maintenance and control of all software. For instance, there should be policies requiring the maintenance of the source code and executable code of each program. In cases where the manufacturer will not release the source code, a source code escrow account should be required. Such an account maintains the program source code to protect both the interests of the health-care facility and the software manufacturer. Should the software manufacturer cease to operate, the source code can be retrieved by the health-care facility. Updates and modifications can then be made as necessary by the health-care facility in the event that the manufacturer goes out of business and can no longer support the product.

Procedures must be put in place to control access to programs and software and to protect them from unauthorized changes, tampering, and damage. Such controls include procedures granting restrictive privileges to individuals for access control for production, audit, and change control purposes. Additionally individuals responsible for the development of software, quality assurance testing, and transferring software to production status should be identified along with specified procedures for carrying out each of these activities.

Access and Other Security Controls

Access control software should be implemented to control individual access to application programs as well as to monitor access to the system. User identification and passwords should be used to log-on computer systems. Passwords should be at least six characters in length and composed of a combination of numeric and alphabetical characters. The combination of alpha and numeric characters makes it harder for an outside intruder to scan systems or to crash into the system through multiple log-on attempts. Passwords should be changed on a regular basis, preferably every 30 to 60 days. Ideally, the password should be automatically generated by the system. This reduces the temptation by employees to use common terms such as spouse name, pet name, and maiden name for their individual passwords. Policies against password sharing should be developed and enforced.

Access to specific applications and files should be limited to a need-to-know basis. In other words, each user has a specific view of the data required to perform his or her job. Delimiting access privileges to databases can be accomplished through the use of appropriate database management software. Access levels should be included in job or position descriptions and employees should be aware of access levels.

At the time of each system access, the system should inform the user of the date and time of the last successful access as well as any unsuccessful log-on attempts. This alerts the user to any unusual activity that may have occurred during the last known successful log-on. If a user suspects that the system was accessed nefariously with his or her log-on ID and password, appropriate organizational security authorities should be notified immediately.

In order to protect the transmission of passwords outside the organizational campus (i.e., use of nondedicated phone lines), passwords and similar authenticators should be obscured by using encryption methods. Encryption is a process by which data are scrambled so that they are made unintelligible to a hacker or invader of the system.

The system should perform a number of other automatic security functions. Among those recommended by the Canada Health Informatics Association are (1995):

- Automatically terminate a user's session after a predetermined period of inactivity. Usually this is within 2 to 3 minutes of inactivity.

- Passwords and similar authenticators should be blocked from appearing on the terminal screen at the time of user log-on.

- A predetermined number of consecutive log-on attempts with invalid passwords should automatically sever the connection with the user and the system. In addition, such an event should send a message to a security administrator or to a log.

- Display screens and all associated memory should be cleared when the user logs off the system or after a predetermined period of inactivity.

- The system should log all transactions automatically, including additions, deletions, or changes to the data. Such a log should be able to recreate a chain of events leading to the data modification.

- Audit trails should be automatically produced and monitored regularly. Automatic alerts, such as multiple unsuccessful log-on attempts, should be generated and routed to the appropriate security personnel.
- Logs for relevant security events should be automatically developed by the system. These events include network-related status messages, computer operator commands and responses, changes to access control information, and changes to lists of authorized users.
- Various integrity controls should be used while data are stored or maintained in the system. Some of these include batch totals, file record counts, hash totals, block counts, and check sums.

Communications Security

With the increased usage of local- and wide-area networks, communications security has become a critical element in security programs. Because of the relative newness of the use of local-area networks and their significant growth, controls and protection of network systems are still evolving. The security management of such networks is a complicated task—many times more complicated than the security of mainframe systems. There are many good texts that address issues involving network security and the student is guided to these and others to study in-depth network security measures (Siyan and Hare, 1995; Shaffer and Simon, 1994).

A network security program should include three primary goals: (1) developing good policy, (2) developing mechanisms for accountability, and (3) developing procedures that implement policy controls. Open systems interconnection (OSI) recommends a security model based on providing five services.

1. *Authentication:* This service ensures that the system knows that the user is authorized.
2. *Access control:* This service controls access to various resources. The access control service relies on the authentication service to accurately identify authorized users.
3. *Data confidentiality:* This service protects data from unauthorized disclosures.
4. *Data integrity:* This service protects against unauthorized modification, insertion, deletion, or replay of all data sets or of selected fields.

5. *Nonrepudiation:* This service prevents individuals from denying that they sent or received communications using the system.

These services are generic in nature. In order to operationalize them, specific mechanisms must be implemented, including the use of encryption, digital signature, access control mechanisms, data integrity mechanisms, authentication exchange, and traffic padding.

Minimally the types of procedures that should be in place for network security include monitoring communication facilities for discrepancies, conducting surveillance tests, and monitoring unsuccessful system access attempts. Whenever data are communicated to remote sites, such as physician offices and laboratories, data should be encrypted. If the health-care organization is connected to public networks such as the Internet, the organizational systems should be protected by use of a firewall. A *firewall* is a set of functions and architecture of devices that protects one network from another. Organizations can either build firewalls internally (usually an expensive alternative) or can purchase off-the-shelf products.

Conclusion

A number of prevention and control countermeasures have been presented. They are discussed in the database and data management chapters and they help the student understand the complexities of data security in the health-care environment. These measures should be systematically implemented in all health-care organizations. New roles in health information management require that the health information manager be knowledgeable with up-to-date skills in assisting in the development and management of a data security program.

Business Continuity Planning

A principal reason for the identification of critical systems and their associated risks is to provide a foundation for the development of a **business continuity plan**. The business continuity plan is sometimes referred to as a disaster plan. The purpose of a business continuity plan is to reduce the impact of an extended system outage on the health-care facility.

There are two major categories of harmful events that can disrupt computer system operation: natural disasters and human-caused disasters. To minimize their impact, the organization should have policies and procedures that provide details on how critical systems will resume after a disastrous event. The management and oversight for the business continuity plan should be given to one individual within the organization. In many cases, the chief security officer is the person responsible for the development and maintenance of the plan. The value of any plan is that it works when required. Therefore, the business continuity plan should be tested periodically. Since hardware and software components of systems change rapidly, it is important that the business continuity plan be reviewed regularly and updated as necessary.

Goals of the Business Continuity Plan

The goal of the business continuity plan is to reduce the duration of the outage of critical information systems. The objective is to be able to resume business operations within an acceptable time frame. It is important to resume normal business operations as quickly as possible in order to maintain customer service and ensure cash flow through the billing and accounts receivable functions.

Usually there are different time frames for resumption of functions of different systems. In the TGL example provided previously, systems with a criticality level of 1 may be targeted to be resumed within 3 days. Other less critical systems may have a more lengthy resumption period, say 7 to 14 days. In any event, most organizations can tolerate up to 3 to 7 days of outage of critical systems. After that period of time, the disruption usually causes major financial or service impacts. The business continuity plan must address every component of critical systems; computer hardware must be restored along with computer programs, data files, and databases.

Development and Content of the Business Continuity Plan

The business continuity plan is based on the information gathered during the risk analysis and assessment. Using these data as the foundation, the following steps must then be completed.

Identification of Minimum Allowable Time Frame for Each System Disruption

Using the criticality and risk levels as a guide, minimum allowable time frames for system disruption are determined for each business function. In some cases, this will be an arbitrary decision. In other cases, where the ALE can be calculated, the organization will have firm data on which to base its decision.

Identification of Internal and External Alternatives for Continuation of Each System

Once the minimum time frames for system disruption are determined, the internal and external alternatives for continuation for each system can be investigated. For example, in cases where a 1–2 day outage is deemed minimal, the organization may have to consider the establishment of a hot site for system backup. A hot site is an auxiliary computer facility, usually located away from the main campus. The hot site is fully operational, running the same configuration, hardware, software, and communications as the health-care facility. In addition, the hot site will have available the most recent backup of data files and databases. For less critical systems, the organization may determine that a cold site is an acceptable alternative. A cold site is usually a computer room that is equipped with communication lines and is ready to receive computer equipment and software a specific number of days after a disaster occurs.

Evaluation of Cost and Feasibility of Each Alternative for Each System

Once the alternatives are identified, they must be evaluated in terms of cost and feasibility. For example, is the yearly lease cost of a hot site really justified from a cost/benefit standpoint? Or is it more practical for the organization to purchase a redundant CPU? Can alternate arrangements be made within the organization to provide the backup capabilities that are necessary? In one university hospital setting, an arrangement was struck with the academic computing center to provide a hot-site backup to the university hospital, and all academic computing would be switched to a cold site should a disaster occur.

Development of Procedures Required to Activate the Plan

Once alternatives have been selected and cost justified, policies and procedures need to be developed to activate the recovery plan. Such procedures will detail when to call a disaster; how specific functions are to be moved to alternative sites or backup facilities; how operations at the backup site will be maintained while the primary site is being restored; and how operations will return to the primary site. The plan must also assign responsibilities for all tasks, identify what vendors or contact persons are to be notified, and outline recovery strategies. The content of a business continuity plan is outlined in Table 9-13.

Table 9-13. Typical Contents of a Business Continuity Plan

1. Introduction and Executive Summary
2. Responsibility for Development and Implementation of the Plan
   2.1. Security management team
   2.2. Emergency operation team
   2.3. Damage assessment team
   2.4. Coordination of implementation
3. Identification of Disaster
   3.1. Identification of the disaster
   3.2. Notification procedures
   3.3. Identification of cause of disaster
   3.4. Communication procedures
4. Recovery Plan by Functional Area
   4.1. Organization and staffing (includes emergency phone numbers)
   4.2. Vendor, contractor, other organization contacts
   4.3. Backup plans for hardware, software applications, system applications, data, and communications
   4.4. Recovery plans for hardware, software applications, system applications, data, and communications
   4.5. Alternate-site contact (name, phone, address)
5. Testing of the Continuity Plan
   5.1. Method of testing plan for each functional area
   5.2. Frequency of testing
6. Appendices

   Includes such essential items as network diagrams; decision matrices; test schedules; vendor emergency contact information; vendor contracts; equipment and software inventories; agreements with alternative vendors and hot and cold sites.

Summary

- Security, audit, and control are critical components in health-care information systems. The health-care data security program must be grounded in fundamental philosophy of recognizing an individual's right to privacy and maintaining the confidentiality of the physician–patient relationship.

- There are three principal goals of a health information security program: (1) protecting the informational privacy of patient-related data, (2) ensuring the integrity of data, and (3) ensuring the availability of information.

- The components of a security program should include a security organizational structure, technological controls, and policies and procedures to meet the requirements of the organization.

- An important part of a security program is the management of risk, including risk analysis and risk assessment.

- Risk analysis entails (1) the identification of threats or risks to security, (2) the measurement of how likely it is that these risks will occur, and (3) the estimation of impact should the harmful event occur.

- Risk assessment determines the organization's vulnerability to threats and establishes the degree of acceptability of system operations.

- The objective of countermeasures is to either (1) prevent a harmful event from occurring or (2) control the damage of the event after it has occurred. Countermeasures can be grouped into the following categories: personnel, physical, hardware, software, and communications security.

- Every security program must include a business continuity plan. The purpose of the business continuity plan is to reduce the impact of an extended system outage.

Review Questions

1. What are the imperatives for the development of national legislation that addresses issues of informational privacy?

2. How can the goals of a security program be operationalized?

3. What are the necessary components of a security program? Why is each component essential?

4. What are the steps in conducting a risk analysis? Are all of these steps essential? Why or why not?

5. What are the minimum countermeasures for each of the following security categories: personnel security; physical security; hardware security; software security; communications security?

6. Discuss the steps in developing a business continuity plan.

Enrichment Activities

Given the following scenario, develop a risk analysis for the clinic and a business continuity plan.

Healthy Risk Clinic is a partnership consisting of 26 partners. The medical practice consists of general internists with some subspecialty representation. During the last 4 to 5 years, the clinic has invested in computer systems and related software and feels well positioned for the managed-care market. The clinic shares the premises with a laboratory company that has numerous labs throughout the state. As part of their agreement with the laboratory company, the practice has a direct terminal link so that the results of their patients' tests can be relayed to the physicians promptly.

As part of an alliance with a local hospital, the clinic is linked with the hospital's computer system through dedicated lines and has been given limited access, for inquiry purposes only, into the following areas:

- Central admitting and registration
- Pharmacy
- Order-entry/results reporting
- Online dictated reporting (i.e., operative, discharge summary, radiology reports)

Recently, the clinic has also provided Internet access to its physicians and managers. The practice has upgraded their computers to 486DX2's operating at 66 megahertz, hard drives 500 MB, 16 MB RAM, and high-quality color monitors. Internal fax/modem boards and CD ROMs are also attached to the personal computers. The system is linked together as a peer-to-peer local-area network. Each of the 26 partners has a PC, the reception/scheduling area has three computers, billing/administration has three computers, and four additional computers are allocated to managers/administration. There is also a PC in the reception area for patient use and patients are encouraged to explore the general health information it contains (and/or Internet) while they are waiting. There are several dumb terminals linked to the laboratory on the premises and can be used to make inquiries about test results for their patients. All the partners have a 486 laptop that they use when they are not in the office. These machines can be used to call into the office network to obtain patient data over regular telephone lines. There are several other pieces of related equipment such as laser printers, a fax machine, and light pens.

Because of the computer growth in the practice and communication links outside the practice, concern has risen about security of the system. You have been contracted as a consultant to perform a threat and risk assessment of the system, recommend a business continuity plan, and make recommendations to safeguard the system in an Internet environment.

The threat and risk assessment should encompass hardware, software applications, data, public domain software, modems, and telecommunications. The threat and risk assessment should provide the basis for the business continuity plan that is developed. Finally, specific recommendations should be highlighted in regard to Internet usage.

The case study above provides sufficient information about the clinic. However, individual assumptions may need to be made. Be sure to note at the beginning of your report any assumptions upon which your recommendations are based.

References

Bialorucki, T., and Blane, M.J. (1992). Protecting patient confidentiality in the pursuit of the ultimate computerized information system. *Journal of Nursing Care Quality, 7* (1), 53–56.

Buck, Edward R. (1991) *Introduction to data security and controls,* 2nd ed. Boston: QED Technical Publishing Group.

COACH—Canada Health Informatics Association (1995). *Security and privacy guidelines for health information systems.* Edmonton, Alberta, Canada: Healthcare Computing and Communications Canada, Inc.

Computer-Based Patient Record Institute, Inc. (1994, April). Position paper: Access to patient data. Chicago, IL.

Dowling, A.F. (1980, Fall). Do hospital staff interfere with computer system implementation? *HCM Review*, pp. 23–32.

Frawley, K.A. (1995, November–December). The Medical Records Confidentiality Act of 1995 introduced. *Journal of the American Health Information Management Association, 66* (10).

Gordon, Mark L., Fogel, Richard L., and McKenzie, Diana J.P. (1993, April). Hospitals protection of patients' records shows strengths and weaknesses. *HIMSS News, 5* (4).

Gostin, L.O., Turek-Brezina, J., Powers, M., and Kozloff, R. (1995, Winter). Privacy and security of health information in the emerging health system. *Health Matrix: Journal of Law-Medicine,* p. 18.

Hafner, K.M., Lewis, G., Kelly, K., Shao, M., Hawkings, C., and Angiolillo, P. (1988, August 1). Is your computer secure? *Business Week,* pp. 64–72.

Hallowell, E.E., and Eldridge, J.E. (1988). The Uniform Health Care Information Act: An informed approach to medical record confidentiality. *Journal of Practical Nursing, 38* (4), 42–45.

Nelson, N.R. (1978). *Computer system integrity, a relative-impact measure of vulnerability.* Menlo Park, CA: Stanford Research Institute.

Privacy Protection Study Commission (1977). Personal privacy in an information society: The report of the Privacy Protection Study Commission. Washington, DC: U.S. Government Printing Office.

Shaffer, Steven L., and Simon, Alan R. *Network security.* Boston, MA: Academic Press.

Siyan, Karanjit, and Hare, Chris (1995). *Internet firewalls and network security.* Indianapolis: New Riders Publishing.

Tipton, Hal (1993). Purposes of information security management. In Zella G. Ruthberg and Harold F. Tipton (eds.), *Handbook of information security management.* Boston: Auerbach.

Wood, Charles Cresson (1993). Organizing the information security function. In Zella G. Ruthberg and Harold F. Tipton (eds.), *Handbook of information security management.* Boston: Auerbach.

In Conclusion

As this textbook was going to press, the American Health Information Management Association had just introduced Vision 2006, the association's vision and definition of professional practice for the next decade. Vision 2006 is a model of professional practice that embraces the concept of information as a corporate asset and is concerned with professional roles that support a suite of information services. These include roles such as clinical data specialist, health information manager, data repository manager, information security officer, patient information coordinator, research and outcomes analyst and data quality manager. Many of these roles are reflected in the professional model of practice presented in Chapter 1.

The knowledge and skill set required to perform many of the Vision 2006 roles significantly departs from that associated with the traditional paradigm of practice. This essentially means a departure from roles as archivists and records managers to those of information management. The intent of this text is to present information management concepts, methods, and techniques which will prepare the student for roles in the design, development, and management of health information in an automated environment. The student, as well as the practitioner, should therefore find this text a useful resource in preparing to meet the challenges of the American Health Information Management Association's Vision 2006.

Glossary

Administrative Information Systems   A group of information system applications such as financial, human resource, materials, and facilities management systems that support the operation and management of an organization.

Annualized Loss Expectancy   The financial impact or loss to the organization should an information system fail.

Attribute   In data modeling, a fact or piece of information about an entity. Also called a field.

Authorization Rules   Rules used to establish the level of access granted to a person, terminal, or program to perform specific operations in an information system.

Bar Chart   A chart that is used to graph nominal data.

Business Continuity Plan   A plan for the emergency recovery of information resources in the event of disaster or system or other failure.

Chief Information Officer (CIO)   An executive-level manager, usually at the vice-presidential level or higher, responsible for enterprise-wide information strategic planning and information resources management.

Chief Security Officer (CSO)   A manager, sometimes at an executive level, who is responsible for enterprise-wide information security management.

Computer-Aided Software Engineering (CASE)   A set of software application tools and programs used in the design, development, and implementation of information systems.

Computer-based Patient Record (CPR)   An electronic patient record that resides in a system specifically designed to support users through availability of complete and accurate data, practitioner reminders and alerts, clinical decision support systems, links to bodies of medical knowledge, and other aids.

Conceptual Data Model   Defines the database requirements of the enterprise in a single database description.

Concurrency Controls   Controls implemented to prevent concurrent updating by two or more individuals of the same data in a database at the same time.

Confidentiality   The expectation that information collected will be used for the purpose for which it was gathered.

Continuous Data Data that can theoretically lie anywhere within a specified interval on a number scale.

Critical Success Factors The limited number of areas in which results, if they are satisfactory, will ensure the successful competitive performance of a business.

Data Noninterpreted items such as facts, images, or sounds that can be processed into useful information.

Data Accuracy Degree of correctness of data.

Data Administrator (DA) Individual responsible for the managerial functions of database administration. Among these functions are planning, policy formulation, database management system evaluation, data dictionary management, and user education.

Data Comprehensiveness Refers to the scope of the data collected.

Data Consistency The degree to which data values for a specific attribute are the same throughout a database.

Data Currency The degree to which data are up to date.

Data Dictionary (DD) A catalog of information about a database including names of records and fields, characteristics about the fields, allowed values for fields, and description of the relationships among entities and application programs that access the database.

Data Granularity Level of detail of attributes and their values.

Data Integrity Consistency and correctness of data throughout a database.

Data Manipulation Language (DML) Commands used by users and application programs to access a database or execute specific database transactions.

Data Modeling Process of determining the data that a business needs and identifying the relationships among these data.

Data Redundancy Duplication of data fields.

Data Relevancy Level of meaningfulness of data to the performance of the process or application for which they are collected.

Data Timeliness The time between the occurrence of an event and the availability of data about that event.

Database Collection of data about entities and their relationship to each other.

Database Administrator (DBA) Manager responsible for both managerial and technical functions of the database administration group.

Database Management System (DBMS) Software system that supports the database approach to data management, providing facilities for the creation, storage, management, access, and protection of data.

Decision Support System (DSS) An information system that consists of interacting dialog, database, and modeling components used to support nonroutine management decisions.

Discrete Data Data that can be plotted on a number scale and that can lie on only certain points and not on the points in between.

Electronic Data Interchange (EDI)   Computer-to-computer interchange of business transactions.

Encryption   Conversion of text into unintelligible form using cryptographic methods.

Entity   A person, place, thing, or concept about which data are gathered.

Entity-Relationship Diagram   A diagram used in the data modeling process that maps out entities and their relationships.

Environmental Analysis   An analysis conducted as part of the strategic planning process that assesses the external environment in which an enterprise exists and usually includes an evaluation of national, political, economic, social, legal, and technological forces.

Executive Information System (EIS)   A type of DSS usually containing an interactive dialog and database component that provides information to senior-level executives for decision-making purposes.

Expert Systems (ES)   An information system that contains a knowledge base, usually restricted to a specific domain, and applies a reasoning methodology and specific rules to provide advice, recommendations, or conclusions to a decision maker.

External Data Model   View of the data by a specific group of users or by a specific processing application.

Feedback   Information flowing from a system output and used to make adjustments or changes in system input or processing activities.

Field   A fact or piece of information about an entity. Also called an attribute.

File   A collection of related records. In a database environment, also called a relation or table.

Frequency Distribution   Display or list, usually in table format, of the number of occurrences of a variable.

Gap Analysis   A step in the strategic planning process that is a structured assessment to identify the discrepancies between the way an organization sees itself and its true position with regard to its competitors and other driving forces in the external environment.

Histogram   A plot of the frequency or percentage distribution.

Hospital Information System   A general description of an organization-wide information system that includes core, business and financial, communications, departmental management, medical documentation, and medical support applications.

Information   Interpreted data or sets of data whose content or form are useful to a particular task.

Information Broker   Professional who acts as an intermediary between a client and information product or group of information services.

Information Engineering   A concept developed by James Martin that takes a holistic view of management of information and employs a development methodology based on four steps: information strategic plan, business area analysis, business system design, and construction.

Information Resources Management (IRM)   A strategy for management of information as an organizational resource including the creation, usage, storage, and eventual disposal of information.

Information System   A group of interrelated and self-adapting components, including people, work procedures, data, and information technologies, working through defined relationships to collect, process, and disseminate data and information for accomplishment of specific organizational goals.

Information Systems Life Cycle   Stages of an information system that include design and development, implementation, operation and maintenance, and obsolescence.

Informational Privacy   The right of individuals to determine at what time, in what way, and to what extent information about them is communicated to others.

In-house system   Information systems that are designed, programmed, supported, and modified by an organization's own information systems staff and that run on computers housed on-site.

Input   The capture, gathering, or collecting of raw data.

Internal Analysis   A step in the strategic planning process that gathers and assesses data to gain an understanding about the way the organization functions and to develop a factual portrait of the organization.

Internal Data Model   Depicts how data are physically represented in a database.

Interval Data   Variables that have the logical and ranking features of ordinal and nominal data but whose categories are defined in terms of a standard unit of measurement.

Joint Application Development (JAD)   Technique used in the process of information system design that brings together in a focused meeting (usually lasting several days) users, analysts, database specialists, programmers, and other interested groups to identify design specifications of an information system.

Knowledge   The application of rules, relationships, and ideas acquired by education or experience.

Laboratory Information System   Information system that supports both the processing of data associated with laboratory tests and management functions associated with day-to-day operations.

Line Graph   A graph that displays the value of the dependent variable for each of several categories on an independent variable.

Management Information System (MIS)   An information system that provides routine information to managers for decision making and planning for the organization.

Mean   The average of a set of values.

Measures of Central Tendency Statistical methods for describing the typical value of a variable.

Measures of Dispersion Statistics that provide data about the spread among individual observations. Among these are the range, standard deviation, and variance.

Median The midpoint or middle-ranking number in a set of values.

Mode The most frequently occurring category or occurring number in a set of values or observations.

Nominal Data Variables that have positively defined categories with no implied distance between one category and the next (e.g., gender, marital status, medical specialty).

Nursing Information System Information system that supports nursing care process from clinical and managerial perspectives.

Office Automation Systems (OAS) Information systems that facilitate day-to-day processing and communication tasks usually including a broad range of tools such as word processors, spreadsheets, database and electronic mail systems.

Ordinal Data Variables that belong to categories that can be ordered or ranked (e.g., upper, middle, low).

Organization-wide Information System Life Cycle A concept developed by Nolan that includes six stages: initiation, expansion, control, integration, data administration, and maturity.

Output Product produced from information systems processes.

Patient Monitoring System Information systems that collect, store, interpret, and display physiologic patient data.

Pharmacy Information System Information system that collects, stores, and manages information related to drugs and the use of drugs in patient care.

Polygon A graph used to plot frequencies and percentages.

Processing Conversion or manipulation of raw data into some useful type of output.

Query by Example (QBE) Data manipulation language that allows the users to easily formulate database queries using structured query screens.

Rapid Application Development (RAD) A set of techniques and tools, including prototyping, CASE tools, screen generators, and report generators, used to speed up the information systems design and development process.

Record A collection of related fields. In a database environment, also called a tuple or row.

Recovery Capacity to restore data, programs, and hardware after the occurrence of system interruption, failure, or destruction.

Request for Proposal (RFP) A formal document used in the selection and evaluation of an information system that is developed by an organization to solicit proposals from information system vendors.

Risk Analysis   A formal assessment of an organization's information assets, controls, and vulnerabilities and determination of the likelihood and potential severity of harmful events and costs should these events occur.

Shared System   Information system that is designed, programmed, and maintained by a system vendor running on computer equipment at the vendor site and shared among a number of vendor clients.

Stand-Alone System   Information systems developed to support a specific set of functional tasks, frequently departmentally based, and which have their own separate application programs, data files, and computer hardware.

Standard Deviation   A measure of dispersion that indicates how far dispersed cases are from the mean.

Statistical Significance Tests   A statistic that indicates the importance of a relationship among variables.

Strategic Planning   An organizational planning process that identifies long-term organizational objectives and associated strategies accomplished by conducting internal and external analyses that assist in identifying future trends, strengths, weaknesses, and opportunities for the organization.

Structured Query Language (SQL)   Data manipulation language that allows users to formulate database queries, manipulate data, and perform various calculations and functions.

SWOT Analysis   A technique used to identify strengths, weaknesses, opportunities, and threats to help an organization assess its current position in relation to the competitive market.

System   A group of components that have the ability to self-adapt and that interact through defined relationships working toward accomplishing a goal.

System Development Life Cycle (SDLC)   Traditional information system development process that includes the four stages of system initiation, development, implementation, and operation.

Transaction Processing System   An information system that collects and stores data about transactions or business-related activities.

Trojan Horse   A computer program used by hackers and other system intruders that masquerades as performing a useful or authorized function but performs additional, malicious functions unknown to the user.

Turnkey System   Information system that usually includes application software and hardware that is not modifiable.

Variance   A statistic that describes how far dispersed cases are from the mean.

Worm   A disruptive and intrusive computer program that reproduces by copying itself from one system to another while traveling from machine to machine over a computer network.

Index

Access patterns, 116
Administrative and management applications, 65–68
  facilities management information systems, 67
  financial information systems, 66
  human resource management information systems, 66
  materials management systems, 66–67
  strategic planning, quality improvement, and decision support, 67–68
Administrative and managerial information systems, 70
AHIMA. *See* American Health Information Management Association
ALE. *See* Annualized loss expectancy
American Health Information Management Association (AHIMA), 5, 260
Analysis of variance (ANOVA), 243
Analyzing data, 228–244
  analysis design, 228–229
  descriptive measures, 232–242
    frequency distribution, 232–233
    measures of association, 239–242
    measures of central tendency, 234–235
    measures of dispersion, 235–239
  determining significance and group differences, 242–244
  fundamental concepts, 230–232
    discrete and continuous data, 231–232
    levels of measurement, 230–231
  sample case data, 230
Annualized loss expectancy (ALE), 277–279
Attribute, 118–119, 152, 162, 197
Authorization controls/rules, 175–176

Bar chart, 247–248, 249
Boar model, 91
Business continuity plan, 294–297
  development and content of, 295–297
  goals of, 295
Business data model, contents of, 114–116

Cartesian coordinate system, 245
CASE tools, 12, 105–107, 119–121, 178
Categories of information systems, 29–31
Chen entity-relationship (ER) style, 116, 117
Chief executive officer (CEO), 79
Chief financial officer (CFO), 79
Chief information officer (CIO), 3–4, 40, 79
Chief operating officer (COO), 79
Chief security officer (CSO), 118, 271, 272
Chi-square test (χ^2), 242
Client, 7–8, 15
Clinical applications and systems, 59–65
  hospital information systems (HIS), 59–62
  laboratory information systems (LIS), 63–64
  nursing information systems (NIS), 63
  patient monitoring systems, 62–63
  pharmacy information systems, 64–65
Clinical information systems, 69
Clinical systems, 54–56
Closed system, 25
CODASYL approach, 163, 165
Code of ethics, 284
Communications security, 293–294
Complex system, 25
Components, information system, 26–27
Computer-aided software engineering (CASE) tools, 12, 105–107, 119–121, 178
Computer-based patient record (CPR), 69, 269
Computer-Based Patient Record Institute (CPRI), 258–259
Computer statistical packages, 253
Concepts of health information management, 18–49
  defining an information system, 20–31
    categories of information systems, 29–31
    information system components, 26–27
    information system concepts, 21–26
    information system processes, 27–28
  importance of systems thinking, 46
  information systems and the organization, 31–46
    impact of information systems technology on the

Concepts of health information management (*cont.*)
  organization, 42–46
    levels of organizational decision making, 32–34
    life cycle of information systems in the organiza-
      tion, 34–38
    managing the information resource, 38–42
    strategic nature of information systems, 31–32
Conceptual data model, 113, 149–150
  contents of, 114–116
Concurrent processing controls, 173–174
Confidentiality, of health data, 258–260
Confidentiality agreement, 285
Continuous data, 231
CPR. *See* Computer-based patient record
Critical success factors (CSF), 83–87
CSF. *See* Critical success factors
Customer, 7–8
Customized information systems planning methodol-
    ogy, 92–96
  development of enterprise-wide information
    model, 94–95
  integration of strategic plans of business informa-
    tion system, 93–94
  top management understanding and support, 92–93
  view of information system as strategic business
    unit, 93

DA. See Data administrator
Data, 52–53, 195
  ensuring availability of, 267
Data accuracy, 199
Data administration, 12
Data administrator (DA), 177
  roles, 177–188
    data dictionary management, 185–187
    DBMS evaluation and selection, 178–185
    planning functions, 178
    security, 187–188
    user training, 187
Database, 157
Database administrator (DBA), 177
  functions, 188–189
Database management systems (DBMS), 157, 159
  evaluation and selection, 178–185
  functions, 168–176
    authorization controls, 175–176
    concurrent processing controls, 173–174
    data dictionary, 170–171
    data integrity services, 172–173
    recovery services, 174–175
    storing, retrieving, and updating, 169–170
    transaction support, 171–172

    user interface, 171
  and promotion of data quality, 207
Databases and their management concepts, 148–191
  database management concepts, 152–168
    database structure models, 159–168
    files, records, and fields, 152–154
    file versus database processing, 154–159
  database management system functions, 168–176.
      See also Database management systems
  functions of data and database administrators,
      176–189
    data administrator roles, 177–188
    database administrator functions, 188–189
Database structure models, 159
  hierarchical model, 167
  network model, 163–166
  object-oriented models, 167–168
  relational model, 160–163
Data comprehensiveness, 198
Data consistency, 199
Data control, 207, 222–224
Data currency, 199
Data dictionary (DD), 170–171
  management of, 185–187
Data flow diagram (DFD), 106
Data granularity, 198
Data integrity, 155
  protection models, 266–267
  services, 172–173
Data manipulation languages (DML), 163
  query by example (QBE), 225–228
  structured query language (SQL), 213–225
Data model diagrams, developing, 128–145
  Martin information engineering style, 129–137
  sample diagram project, 137–145
  translation of conceptual model to physical model,
      145
Data modeling, 12, 108–110
  definition of, 111–112
  methods and styles, 116–119
  steps in modeling process, 119–128
    formation of team, 119
    selection of tools, 119–121
    defining user requirements, 121–127
    documenting data flows, uses, and requirements,
      128
Data models, categories of, 113
  conceptual, 113
  external, 113
  internal, 113
Data quality, managing, 192–210
  characteristics of data quality, 196–200

determining the quality of data, 200–207
   analyzing results of monitoring and tracking, 206
   determining data quality requirements, 201–204
   implementing information systems data control
      features, 207
   improving processes that use and create data,
      206–207
   measuring and tracking data quality, 204–206
   origins of data quality, 195–196
Data redundancy, 155
Data relevancy, 196–197
Data representation, 200
Data retrieval and analysis, 155, 211–255
   analyzing data, 228–244. *See also* Analyzing data
   data presentation techniques, 244–253
      graphing data, 244–252
      use of computer statistical packages, 253
   retrieval and manipulation of data, 213–228
      query by example (QBE), 225–228
      structured query language (SQL), 213–225
Data timeliness, 198–199
DBA. *See* Database administrator
Decision-making levels, 32–34
Decision support systems (DSS), 30, 57, 58, 68
Descriptive measures, 232–242
   frequency distribution, 232–233
   measures of association, 239–242
   measures of central tendency, 234–235
   measures of dispersion, 235–239
Design and development of information systems,
      100–147
   developing data model diagrams, 128–145
      Martin information engineering style, 129–137
      sample data modeling diagram project, 137–145
      translation of conceptual data model to physical
         data model, 145
   new approaches and new tools, 104–108
      computer-aided software engineering tools,
         105–107
      development of enterprise information model,
         104–105
      joint application design, 108
      rapid application development tools, 107–108
   traditional systems development life cycle, 101–104
   use of new approaches for analysis and design,
      108–128
      categories of data models, 113–114
      contents of conceptual or business data model,
         114–116
      data modeling, 108–110
      data modeling methods and styles, 116–119
      definition of data modeling, 111–112
      steps in data modeling process, 119–128
Diagnostic-related groups (DRGs), 57–58
Diagrams, 114–115
Discontinuity, 36
Discrete data, 231
Downloaded files, 264–265
Dynamic system, 26

Edit checks, 173
Electronic data interchange (EDI), 269
Encryption, 176
Enterprise information model, development of,
      104–105
Enterprise strategy, developing, 88
Entity, 117, 152, 197
Entity-relationship diagram (ERD), 104, 106
Environmental analysis, 81–83
Executive information systems (EIS), 30, 57, 58
Expert systems (ES), 30, 57
External data model, 113

Facilitator, 79–80
Facilities management information system, 67
Feedback, 24, 28
Field, 153
File, 153
File processing, 154–155
Financial information systems, 54–55, 66
Fire protection, 287–288
Firewall, 294
Frequency distribution, 232–233
Frequency polygon, 248–249, 250
F-statistic test, 242, 243–244

Gap analysis, 85
Glossary, 115
Graphing data, 244–252
   distortions in graphing, 250–251
   frequency polygon, 248–249, 250
   histogram, 246–248
   line graph, 249–250, 252
Group decision support software (GDSS), 127

Hardware security, 288–289
Health-care organizational strategic planning process,
      78–88
   environmental and internal analyses, 81–88
      environmental analysis, 81–83
      internal analysis, 83–85
      summary paper preparation, 88
   organizing resources, 79–81
      development of task groups, 81

Health-care organizational strategic planning
     process, (*cont.*)
  hiring a facilitator, 79–80
  other resources, 80
  planning team, 79
Health information, 9
Health information management, xviii-xx
  concepts of, 18–49
  definitions of, xi, 3–8
  model of practice, 1–17
Health information manager
  as information broker, 7-8
  as marketer of services, 14–15
  model of practice, 9–14
  role in strategic IS planning, 97
Health maintenance organizations (HMOs), 58
Hierarchical database model, 167
HIS. *See* Hospital information systems
Histogram, 245, 246–248
HMO. *See* Health maintenance organizations
Hospital information systems (HIS), 59–62
Human resource management information systems,
     66

Information, 53
Informational privacy models, 265–266
information analysis, 13–14
Information engineering (IE), 9, 10–12, 76, 77
  data administration, 12
  data modeling, 12, 116, 117
  process modeling, 12
  report design, 12
  screen design, 12
  strategic planning, 11–12
Information life cycle of the organization, 36–38
Information management (IM), traditional definitions
     of, 3–4
Information resources management (IRM), 3, 38–42,
     70
  concepts of, 39–40
  evolution of information systems, 38–39
  information resources management organization,
     40–42
Information retrieval, 12–13
Information systems
  categories of, 29-31
  components, 26–27
  concepts, 21–26
  defining, 20–31
  design and development, 100–147
  in health care, 50–74
  and the organization, 31–46

  processes, 27–28
  strategic planning for, 75–99
Information systems life cycle (ISLC), 35
Information system types, 57–59
In-house developed systems, 56
Inputs, 24, 27
Internal analysis, 83–85
Internal data model, 113
Interval data, 230
Interval variables, 230–231

Joint application design (JAD), 103, 108, 126
Joint Commission on Accreditation of Health Care
     Organizations (JCAHO), 188

Knowledge, 53–54

Laboratory information systems (LIS), 63–64
Length of stay (LOS), 228–229
Levels of organizational decision making, 32–34
Life cycle of information systems, 34–38
Line graph, 245, 249–250, 252
Local-area network (LAN), 59
LOS. *See* Length of stay

Management information systems (MIS), 30, 57, 58
Martin information engineering method, 129–137
  IE concepts and methods of notation, 130–137
  stages of the method, 129–130
Materials management systems, 66–67
Mean, 232, 234–235
Measures of association, 239–242
Measures of central tendency, 234–235
Measures of dispersion, 235–239
Median, 232, 234–235
Medical documentation systems, 61–62
Medical record professionals, traditional roles of, 5–6
Mode, 232, 234–235
Model of practice for health information management
  definitions of health information management, 3–8
    health information manager as information
       broker, 7–8
    requirements of role change, 6–7
    traditional definitions of information manage-
       ment, 3–4
    traditional roles of medical record professionals,
       5–6
  model of practice, 9–14
    information analysis, 13–14
    information engineering domain, 10–12
    information retrieval domain, 12–13
    policy development, 14

successful health information manager, 14–15
Multivariate analysis of variance (MANOVA), 244

Narratives, 115
Network database model, 163–166
Nijssen's information analysis methodology (NIAM), 116
Nominal data, 230, 234
Nominal variables, 230–231
Normal distribution, 236
Nursing information systems (NIS), 63

Object-oriented database models, 167–168
Office automation systems (OAS), 30, 57
Open system, 25–26
Operational decision making, 33
Options, generating, 88
Ordinal data, 234
Ordinal variables, 230–231
Organization-wide information systems life cycle, 35
Outputs, 24, 28

Passwords, 291–292
Patient monitoring systems, 62–63
Percentage polygon, 248–249, 251
Permanent system, 26
Personnel security, 284–286
    change in job function or termination, 285
    corrective or disciplinary action, 286
    security procedures in employee hiring, 284–285
Pharmacy information systems, 64–65
Physical data model, 149–152
Physical security, 286–288
    fire, utilities, and other protections , 287–288
    physical access, 287
    physical location, 286–287
Planning team, 79
Policy development, 14
Polygon, 245, 248–249, 250, 251, 252
Presentation techniques, 244–253
    graphing data, 244–252
    use of computer statistical packages, 253
Privacy Act of 1974, 261
Privacy of health data, 258–260
    legislative protection of, 260–262
Processes, information system, 27–28
    feedback, 28
    input, 27
    output, 28
    processing data, 27–28
Processing mechanisms, 24, 27–28

Process modeling, 12
Professional Practice Standards (AHIMA), 5

QBE. *See* Query by example
Query by example (QBE), 225–228

RADT system. *See* Registration–admission–discharge–transfer system
Range, 235
Rapid application development (RAD) tools, 103, 107–108
Ratio variables, 231
Record, 153
Recovery services, 174–175
Registration–admission–discharge–transfer (RADT) system, 60–61, 268
Relational database model, 160–163
Relations, 160, 162
Relationships, 152–154
Report design, 12
Request for proposal (RFP), 180–185
    RFP documents, 180–184
    RFP process, 185–186
Retrieval and manipulation of data, 213–228
    query by example (QBE), 225–228
    structured query language (SQL), 213–225
RFP. *See* Request for proposal
Risk analysis and management, 274–283
    development of countermeasures, 282–283
    risk analysis, 275–280
        evaluating information assets, 277–279
        identification of assets, 276–277
        risk analysis methods, 279–280
    sample risk assessment, 280–282
Risk assessment, 274–275, 280–282

Schema, 159
Screen design, 12
SDLC. *See* Systems development life cycle
Security, audit, and control of health data, 256–301
    business continuity planning, 294–297
        development and content of plan, 295–297
        goals of plan, 295
    establishing security plan, 268–274
        components of security plan, 270–273
    legislative protection of privacy, 260–262
    prevention and control countermeasures, 283–294
        communications security, 293–294
        hardware security, 288–289
        personnel security, 284–286
        physical security, 286–288
        software security, 289–293

Security, audit, and control of health data (*cont.*)
  privacy and confidentiality of health data, 258–260
  risk analysis and management, 274–283
    development of countermeasures, 282–283
    risk analysis, 275–280
    sample risk assessment, 280–282
  security fundamentals, 262–268
    ensuring data availability, 267
    protecting data integrity, 266–267
    protecting informational privacy, 263–266
Security program, establishing, 268–274
  components of, 270–273
    determining scope, 270–271
    organization, 271–273
    policies, procedures, and standards, 273
Shared systems, 56
Simple system, 24–25
Software security, 289–293
  access and other security controls, 291–293
  control of software, 290–291
  purchase of software, 290
  software development life cycle, 289–290
SQL. *See* Structured query language
Stable system, 26
Stand-alone systems, 57
Standard deviation, 232, 236–239
Standards development, 70–71
Statistical significance, 242–244
Strategic alignment modeling (SAM), 90
Strategic decision making, 32
Strategic nature of information systems, 31–32
Strategic planning, 11–12, 78
Strategic planning in information systems, 75–99
  health-care organizational strategic planning
      process, 78–88
    environmental and internal analyses, 81–88
    generating options and developing an enterprise
        strategy, 88
    organizing resources, 79-81
  health information manager's role in strategic IS
      planning, 97

information system strategic planning, 89–97
    developing customized information systems
        planning methodology, 92–96
    information system strategic planning methods,
        89–92
Structured query language (SQL), 213–225
  data control, 222–224
  data definition: creating database, 214–220
  data manipulation: updating database, 221–222
Subschema, 159
SWOT (strengths, weaknesses, opportunities, and
    threats) analysis, 85–87
System
  characteristics, 21–23
  classification of, 24
  defined, 21
  elements, 24
Systems development life cycle (SDLC), 101–104
Systems thinking, importance of, 46

Tactical decision making, 32–33
Task groups, 81
Temporary system, 26
Transaction processing systems (TPS), 30, 57
Transaction support, 170–171
Trojan horses, 265
T-test of significance, 242–243
Tuple, 162
Turnkey systems, 56–57

Unauthorized user activity, 264
Uniform Health Care Information Act, 261
User interface, 171
User requirements, defining, 121–127
User training, 187

Variance, 235–236
Virtual health care information system, 71

Worm, 267